AMANDA FLETCHER

Fitness Guide For Senior Women 60+

Ditch the Gym, Embrace Fun Workouts! Overcome stiffness, low energy, and mood swings with simple, enjoyable strength and balance exercises to boost confidence!"

Copyright © 2025 by Amanda Fletcher

All rights reserved. No part of this publication may be reproduced, stored or transmitted in any form or by any means, electronic, mechanical, photocopying, recording, scanning, or otherwise without written permission from the publisher. It is illegal to copy this book, post it to a website, or distribute it by any other means without permission.

Amanda Fletcher asserts the moral right to be identified as the author of this work.

Amanda Fletcher has no responsibility for the persistence or accuracy of URLs for external or third-party Internet Websites referred to in this publication and does not guarantee that any content on such Websites is, or will remain, accurate or appropriate.

Designations used by companies to distinguish their products are often claimed as trademarks. All brand names and product names used in this book and on its cover are trade names, service marks, trademarks and registered trademarks of their respective owners. The publishers and the book are not associated with any product or vendor mentioned in this book. None of the companies referenced within the book have endorsed the book.

The information in this book is for general informational and educational purposes only and is not a substitute for professional advice, diagnosis, or treatment. Always seek the advice of your physician or other healthcare professionals with any questions you may have regarding your current health status or a medical condition before starting any fitness activity in this book.

First edition

This book was professionally typeset on Reedsy.
Find out more at reedsy.com

To my husband, Paul—my unwavering source of support, motivation, and inspiration. Your dedication to setting and achieving goals, both in life and as a champion runner, continues to amaze me. Thank you for always being by my side, and cheering me on every step of the way.

To my children, Sunny, Sebastian, and Morgan—you are my greatest joy and my constant reminders of love, strength, and resilience.

With Love Always

Amanda xxx

"It is not the years in your life that count.
It's the life in your years."

-Abraham Lincoln

Contents

Foreword	ii
Preface	iv
Acknowledgments	vi
About This Book	viii
Introduction	xi
Age Is Just a Number, Darling!	xxviii
Stretching the Truth (and Your Hamstrings)	lii
Bone-anza! Keeping Those Bones Strong	lxxv
Cardio, Finding Your Groove-Keep Your Heart Happy	lxxxiii
Yoga, Pilates, and Pretzel-Like Positions	xcvi
Strength Training for Senior Superwomen	cvii
The Art of Falling Gracefully (and Avoiding It)	cxv
Food, Glorious Food! Eating for Energy and Vitality	cxxiv
Dressing the Part: Workout Gear or Glam Gear?	cxxxviii
Workout Buddies: From Friends to Furry Companions	cli
Tech and Tracksuits: Embracing Fitness Gadgets	clxvii
Rest Days and Naps: The Real MVPs	clxxvii
Laughing Through It All-The Power of Humor After 60+	clxxxvii
Your Fitness Legacy: Inspiring the Next Generation	cc
About the Author	2

Foreword

Foreword
 By Rev. Dr. Warren B. Leigh

It is a rare privilege to witness a person channel their unique gifts, experiences, and wisdom into something that has the potential to transform lives. Amanda Fletcher has done exactly that with *Fitness Guide for Senior Women Over 60*. In these pages, she offers not just a guide but a lifeline—a roadmap for women seeking vitality, purpose, and a renewed sense of self in their golden years.

Amanda is an extraordinary woman whose life epitomizes resilience, determination, and balance. An accomplished endurance athlete, Masters GB international competitor, and creator of transformational retreats, Amanda's journey is proof that age is not a limitation but an invitation to thrive. Her deep connection to nature, spirituality, and the holistic principles of fitness has allowed her to develop an approach that blends physical strength with emotional and spiritual well-being—a rare and beautiful harmony.

What sets this book apart is Amanda's ability to connect deeply with her audience. She writes with the compassion of someone who has walked the same path, navigating the challenges of menopause, self-doubt, and the quest for purpose. Her voice is authentic, her wisdom hard-earned, and her advice both practical and profound. Whether you are a seasoned fitness enthusiast or someone just beginning to explore what your next chapter could look like, you will find encouragement and actionable steps here.

This guide is important because it addresses a critical yet often overlooked truth: life does not end at 60—it begins anew. In a society that often sidelines older women, Amanda reminds us that there is no expiration date on joy, adventure, and personal transformation. She offers not only practical tools for achieving physical health but also inspiration for nurturing the mind and spirit.

On a personal note, I have had the privilege of witnessing Amanda's journey during the time we have known each other as a decisive action taker and coordinator. Her energetic presence, unwavering determination, and intuitive understanding of others have always struck me as extraordinary. She brings these qualities to this book with an open heart and a clear vision. Reading it is akin to sitting down with a trusted friend who believes in your potential even when you might doubt it yourself.

As you turn these pages, prepare to be inspired, challenged, and uplifted. Amanda's words are not merely instructions; they are an invitation to rediscover yourself, to embrace the possibilities that lie ahead, and to live the life you truly deserve.

With gratitude and admiration,
   Rev. Dr. Warren B. Leigh

Preface

When I first embarked on my fitness journey decades ago, I never imagined it would lead me to this moment—writing a book to inspire senior women to reclaim their health, confidence, and joy. Over the years, I've experienced firsthand the transformative power of movement, not just in building strength but in nurturing resilience, confidence, and a deeper connection to life itself.

The idea for this book grew out of countless conversations with women who felt lost in the demands of life or disconnected from their sense of purpose. Many longed for practical advice and a sense of hope—a belief that it's never too late to rewrite your story. I've walked this path myself, overcoming physical and emotional challenges, and it's deeply fulfilling to now share these lessons with others.

This book is a blend of everything I've learned as an athlete and woman navigating her 60s with energy and optimism. As a retreat leader over the years, it has enabled me to see the results of my programs every week. My guests would warm to living exactly how I live in my home, training, and helping to cook healthy meals. An up close and personal fitness coach for mind, body, and soul. All issues and worries could be discussed as they arose during guest stays. This has enabled me to chapter the book addressing all the key issues and concerns I discovered from my guest that repeated to form patterns.

This allowed me to provide a wealth of valuable information and activities tailored to their needs and goals, all delivered in a relaxed, natural setting—completely free of the rigidity of traditional classrooms. It's my way of offering encouragement, tools, and a reminder that fitness and self-discovery are gifts we can embrace at any age.

I invite you to step into this journey with me—to discover how much more vibrant, capable, and alive you truly are. Let's make this a new beginning filled with strength, purpose, and joy.

Acknowledgments

Acknowledgments

Writing this book has been a deeply personal and fulfilling journey, and I am forever grateful to the incredible people who have shaped and inspired me along the way.

You have been my greatest teachers to the many remarkable women who attended my retreats over the years. I have learned so much through your courage, resilience, and willingness to embark on transformative journeys. Although I cannot name you individually, know that your stories and growth are the foundation of this book.

To my dear friends, who have been endless sources of humor, wisdom, and support—you've given me countless moments to reflect on and plenty of inspiration to write about.

To my husband, Paul, my rock and motivator—your unwavering support and belief in me have been my driving force. Thank you for being my champion, running partner, and constant source of love and inspiration.

To my children, Sunny, Sebastian, and Morgan, and our five wonderful cats—thank you for filling my life with love, laughter, and endless joy.

And to the Mikkelson twins, Ramus and Christian, your dedication to coaching and guiding me through this publishing process has been invaluable. Thank you for giving me the tools and confidence to bring my vision to life.

Finally, to my readers, thank you for picking up this book and trusting me to be a part of your journey. May you find inspiration, strength, and joy in these pages as you enter the vibrant, empowered life you deserve.

With deep gratitude,
　Amanda Fletcher xxx

About This Book

Welcome to **Fitness Guide for Senior Women 60+,** a refreshing and empowering resource designed to inspire women over 60 to embrace their golden years with renewed vigor, confidence, and joy. The book is based on my experiences and those of my retreat guests of a similar age to myself now 64, from total beginners to those with a reasonable level of fitness seeking guidance, purpose, and rebalance. Whether starting your fitness journey or rediscovering your passion for a healthy lifestyle, this book is your road map to aging gracefully, with strength and vitality.

Think of this as your witty, wisdom-packed, workout buddy that doesn't make you wake up at 5 a.m. or give a frown when you skip leg day.

Inside, you'll find a combination of humor, wisdom, and practical advice to transform how you approach fitness, nutrition, and personal growth at 60 and beyond. From easy-to-follow workouts to heartfelt anecdotes, this book celebrates the idea that age is just a number—and it's never too late to write your next chapter.

If you are not keen on the gym and it fills you with dread, worry not because I'm not keen either, and 'my gym' of Amanda is everywhere and it's free Summer or Winter, discover how here. This book solves many issues and concerns over time and travel. Yes, learn how to do it all in one easy go on the go!

Whether you're dusting off your trainers or discovering them for the first time, this book offers practical exercises, motivational tips, and a generous sprinkle of humor to remind you: that fitness can be fun, fabulous, and doable at any age. Let's laugh, stretch, and strengthen through the golden years together!

A Holistic Approach to Fitness and Health

Explore my customized workout routines, practical nutrition strategies, and mindfulness exercises tailored specifically for women over 60. If you want to stay active, regain flexibility, or boost your confidence, every chapter is designed to meet your needs at your own pace. I have based my activities on what has worked for me on these pages. I am now mindful of my rest days; and not skipping them as in my younger race training days, because I felt great that day. I truly understand past 60, rest days are vital to feel fabulous for the next full fitness day. My days in between will always include a walk for one hour or more. That way I know I have been active in a gentle way in nature, even if that requires an umbrella!

Building a New Mindset and Lifestyle

Discover how to set realistic goals, plan exciting new adventures, and reignite your zest for life. Exploring travel inspiration, hobby ideas, and motivational stories, you'll identify how to create a fulfilling life full of energy, exploration, and self-discovery.

"It's never too late to be what you might have been."
— **George Eliot**

This book is more than a guide—it's your companion on a journey to celebrate the vibrant, confident, and unstoppable version of yourself who's waiting to shine. Let's step into this chapter together!

Introduction

My name is Amanda Fletcher, almost 65, (63 in the photo!), married with three grown-up children who've left home. We live in Manchester, England. I am an author passionate about health, wellness, and fitness, focusing on empowering women and especially seniors as one myself now, through my experiences and humor.

I have and always will lead by my example. I am drawing my background and from over 17 years as a creator and guide of yoga and running retreats for women seeking a total life change from being overweight, having health issues, and lacking any fitness at all starting as beginners to burnt-out corporate women in Spain.

I consider myself an accomplished endurance trail athlete, winner of many races, and have competed internationally for Masters Team GB. I use my knowledge gained and expertise in mindful training combining diet, running, and the benefits of yoga.

In 2017, I opened my first-ever music and yoga festival in Spain. A huge achievement I never dreamt possible with international stars of the music and yoga world performing.

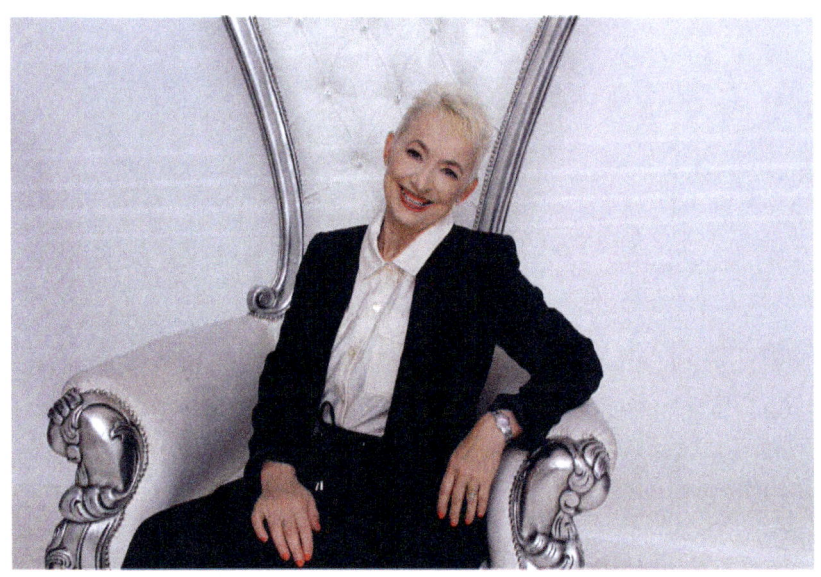

Amanda Fletcher

Welcome

Hello, Welcome.

My primary audience is women aged 60 and above, seeking inspiration for transformative living. My writing reflects a mix of personal and retreat guest struggles with goals and successes achieved. I have always been a very spiritual person, a truth seeker which has heightened since my conscious awakening in 2012, with a lifelong love for storytelling. Finally, since 2012, my spiritual journey of consciousness, it is time to put pen to paper to allow me to guide more ladies worldwide. My husband has encouraged me to write this book. A challenging task with

5 rescue cats who adore sitting on my shoulder, or lap, or demanding food.

A beautiful lady and actress once said
  "Each age has its special joys and experiences. It's up to us to find them."
  — **Audrey Hepburn**

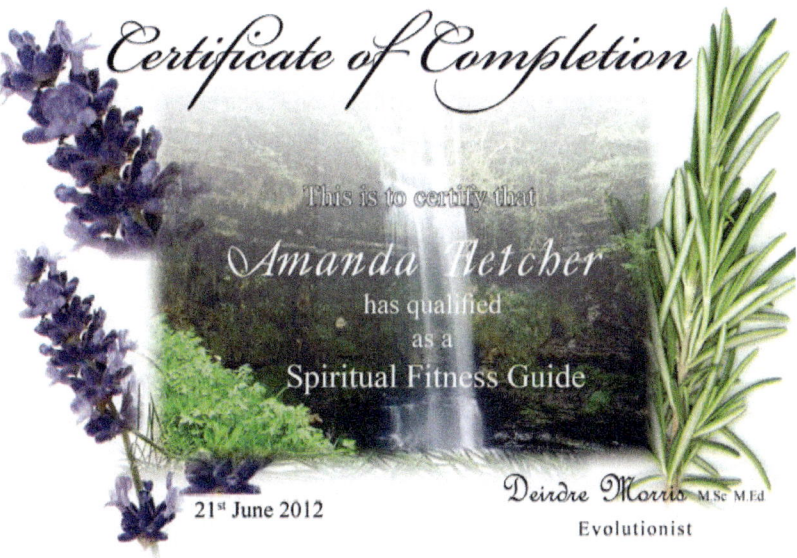

As a **certified Spiritual Fitness Guide** since 2012, a program collaboration with Deirdre Morris, my mentor on my spiritual fitness journey, who opened my mind onto a conscious path, an amazing lady and author who's since collaborated with Jack Canfield on a book together. I am thankful to her for all her encouragement to write my book since we first met in 2012. I've dedicated myself to helping women rediscover their vitality and confidence, particularly in their golden years.

Through decades of experience in health, fitness, and wellness, I've witnessed the many struggles women face as they navigate the demands of career, family, and well-being. Fitness often becomes the first casualty of this balancing act, pushed to the back burner for far too long.

Struggles Older Women Face

For many women, the meaning of life and a wake-up call comes around age 50. Subtle weight gain, persistent fatigue, feeling a sense of being overwhelmed. As children leave the nest and the whirlwind of career and family life settles, these women often find themselves at a crossroads. After years of planning for their needs and families, they suddenly realize they forgot to plan the next chapter of their lives. For some, it's a loss of confidence outside their roles as office professionals or homemakers.

For others, who may have sacrificed partnerships, marriage, or even the chance to have children, it's a profound question of identity and purpose.

This sense of loss, while powerful, can also be a pivotal moment, a chance to reclaim life, discover new passions, and embrace fitness and well-being in ways they may never have imagined. I've had the privilege of guiding countless women on this journey through retreats and personal coaching. Many found love, purpose, and joy again, whether by moving to new countries, starting happy marriages post-50, or simply reconnecting with themselves. The heartfelt emails I've received from these women, who transformed their lives, are a testament to the resilience and potential we all carry within us, no matter our age.

This **Fitness Guide for Senior Women Over 60** is my way of sharing that journey with you, offering the tools, encouragement, and inspiration to take control of your health and happiness in this vibrant chapter of life.

My greatest reward has always been using my divine intuition and practical skills, honed during my career-driven life, to offer useful and spiritual solutions to others. I've learned that mindset is the foundation of any transformation. It starts with resetting goals, focusing on what truly matters, and manifesting those goals through consistent action. Combined with fitness, dietary, and menopausal changes; areas we often neglect, this holistic approach creates powerful shifts to rebalance overall wellbeing.

Our bodies are incredible machines, powered by water and electrical energy, and how we fuel them affects every aspect of how we feel and function. During my retreats, guests would embrace the same lifestyle I live, and within just 10 days, they'd leave with a renewed sense of purpose, a fitness plan, and excitement to embark on their next chapter. When my guests arrived feeling burned out and some in tears of joy and relief to step off their merry-go-round of career and lifestyle choices to let go and leave transformed, with new goals and a fresh outlook on life, was rewarding for me to witness firsthand.

Many ladies believed yoga was the "magic fix" for all their struggles, a 10-day retreat was the solution before returning home, and re-balance was the key. By combining yoga, fitness, and spirituality, I created a space where they could relax, rediscover their passions, and release long-held emotional burdens. Meditative walks, gentle weight loss, and a kick-start to their fitness journey were all part of the experience. Just simply letting it all go in a safe place.

For many women, the early signs of menopause sneak up quietly, often unnoticed, only to hit hard later. Around 54, I began experiencing night sweats. As a seasoned runner, I thought, "No big deal, I'm tough, I can handle this!" But it started to impact my running. When I asked other women runners my age about it, I was surprised by how taboo the topic seemed, more so than discussing cancer! Some women told me to take hormone replacement therapy (HRT),(hormone replacement therapy), but as someone who lives naturally, that was never an option for me. I just sucked it up and pushed on.

There comes a time when it's not failing to reach out to another to ask for help; exactly what I did. I sought the help of a Naturopath called Ella, who quickly put me back onto a successful path. I was fired up planning a half marathon in 12 weeks, I was back rearing to go as I had done in my 50s.

After years of trial and error, I sought help. A doctor confirmed I was out of hormones, and while HRT was suggested, he also recommended exploring natural solutions. I adjusted my diet and experimented with vitamins and minerals, it wasn't until I visited a naturopath who used a frequency diagnostic machine that everything changed. With a tailored plan of supplements, my physical symptoms disappeared. Now, at nearly 65, I feel better than I did in my 40s or 50s!

We don't notice how aging affects us when we're caught up in life's demands. For me, running had become a struggle, but persistence and seeking help turned everything around. My first lesson for you is this: never be afraid to ask for help. Trust your intuition. As women, we're taught to stay strong, but over time, that "strength" can wear us down physically, mentally, and emotionally.

Thinking of a New Life Plan

Aging doesn't mean giving up on yourself. Whether it's tackling new fitness goals, resetting your diet, or even navigating the latest tech (yes, my kids have become my teachers on that front!), it's all possible. If I can overcome the hurdles of menopause, technology, and shifting priorities, so can you. Together, we'll fill in the missing parts of your life, help you set and achieve meaningful goals, and embrace this incredible chapter ahead. To make life changes you must first decide what your dreams, goals, and desires are for the next chapter and write them down in your journal to look back on later.

There is no magic wand treatment, I would always tell my guests. Change starts with you!

"Do one thing every day that scares you."
— **Eleanor Roosevelt**

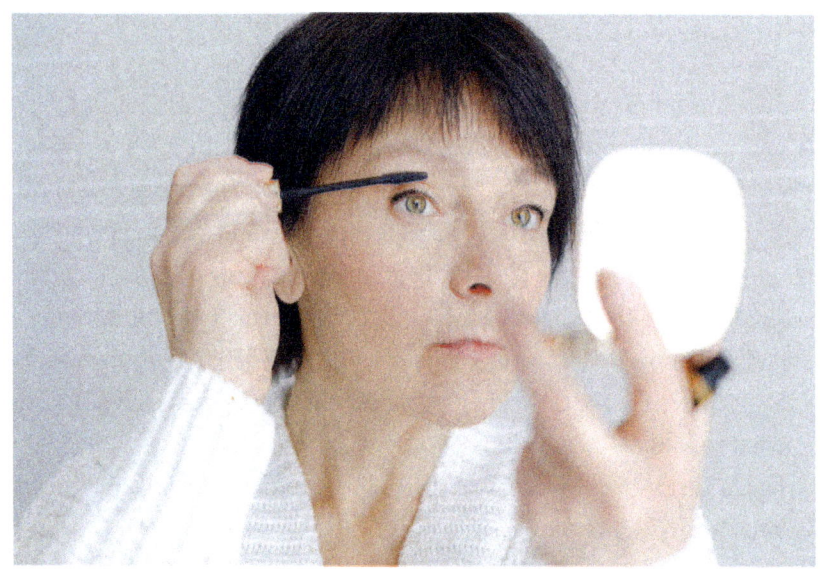

Make-Up on Are You Ready?

I realized many years ago we learn from everyone in our lives and those who touch it.

My goal with my book for you is to find motivation and takeaway inspiration on the pages to start the next chapter of your life to share with others.

This is what my most recent from zero to hero senior had to say about me and my guidance for her decision to run a half marathon in Marrakesh Morocco with 12 weeks to train!

"Dearest Amanda, I am so grateful for you! All of you, not just the bits of me! I have learned so much already and this is just the beginning. Just wanted to send you a small token of my appreciation and to let you know that I think you're fab! Lots of Love Aseea" xxx

Who has become a good friend, and we bonded immediately with the same passions and interests. We met via booking a room at her gorgeous AirBB near London, whilst I was attending a course at the airport.

I am so glad you are reading this book, you have already taken the first step to seek help, your mindset first. I aim to inspire and motivate you too, with plenty of fun treats for fitness throughout this book, along with strengthening and helping you live an amazing big bold strong life.

Enjoy reading and learning some new tricks and tips. I would be honored if you could spend a few minutes to leave me a review for others to find inspiration and new motivation 60+ in their lives too.

Dedication to my Special Senior Friends

For my amazing husband, whom I love dearly, who is always there for me no matter what I want to achieve, who never fails to encourage and inspire me, and for his patience and providing copious mugs of tea to allow me to sit down and write this book. He's my superhero for fitness, training, and mindset goal achievement and now an international gold medalist Masters champion in 2019 Venice at 61, now 66 in training for the World event. We never stop goal setting and targets to aim for, we don't have to nor should we.

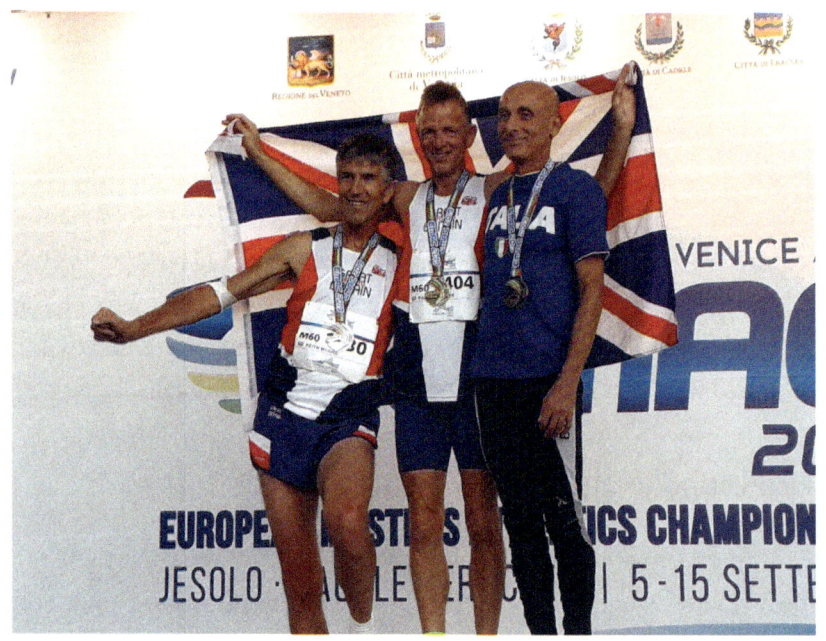

"The only one who can tell you ' you can't' is you. And you don't have to listen." -Nike

'There is no secret in the world that cannot be discovered, once you are ready to listen. The air carries memory and knowledge. All you have to do is just breathe it in.'

~ The Seventh Magpie By Lesley Anne Sharrock

Lesley, a stranger and a new guest booked to stay with me to get fit and healthy for three weeks. As an author, while writing her latest book in between her fitness training and classes, Lesley wanted to combine writing with fitness whilst someone else took care of the program and diet. Seeking to find inspiration in a peaceful location to write, she requested to attend by herself as my only guest. Lesley loved the location in Spain, so much so she never went home!

We quickly became friends and Lesley had already decided this part of Spain was to be her new home. She was always the light and soul of any evening. I would always call her and her partner Ian another beautiful soul, 'time bandits'. I noticed any time spent with them went into warp speed with all their life knowledge and research as writers and publishers. They both taught me about putting pen to paper. Lesley would often say Amanda come on and write a book. They both inspired me, and I definitely would as soon as possible write about my achievements with fitness guests to inspire others.

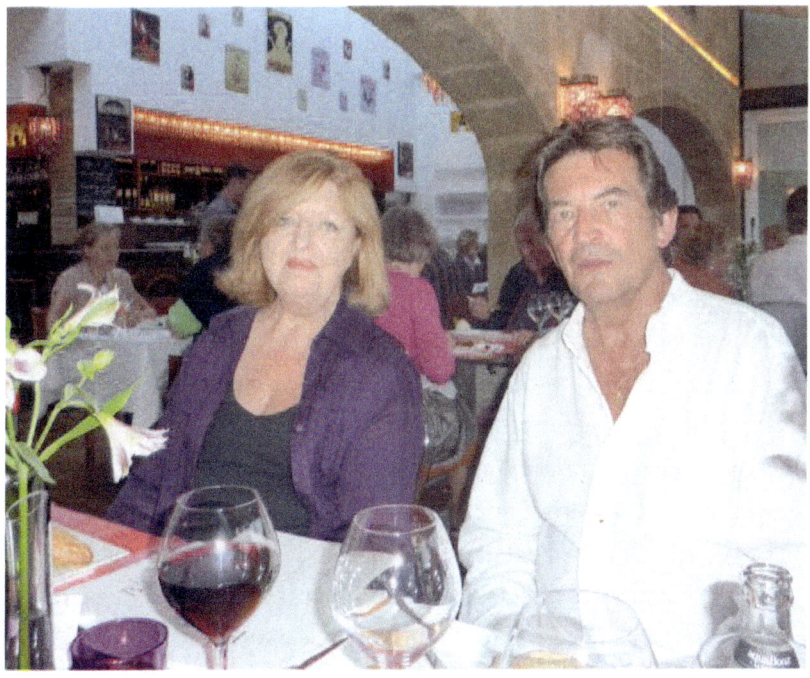

Authors Lesley and Ian

The world pandemic got in the way of my business. Sadly Lesley passed too soon just before the lockdown suddenly and Ian followed not long after during the lockdown. They left a huge void in my life.

I miss them very much, but writing this book I feel they are looking over my shoulder helping me from spirit.

Retreat review

"Dear Amanda, Thank you for a great time, hard work, but rewarding. I can certainly feel the difference already! I will be back to show the progress I have made. A journey of a thousand miles may begin with the first step, but this was more like a leap in the right direction with your program." Thanks Again Sarah B

For me, I hear them say age is just a number, but let's be real it's also a reason some of us groan a little louder when getting off the couch! I am on a new course to seek the best diet and health for my age. The wake-up call comes consciously one day and every day is very precious. Perhaps you are thinking about retiring and need new goals that may include travel and activities. Contained in *Fitness Guide For Senior Women 60+* is here to prove that those groans don't define you and that getting older can mean getting stronger, livelier, and, yes, even sassier!

This isn't your granddaughter's TikTok workout plan. No, it's a collection of simple, effective routines tailored to fit your pace and lifestyle, and, most importantly, your sense of humor to laugh at yourself is wonderful. To learn it doesn't matter, it's a life program, so get back up and start again the next day, but laugh at the best free medicine going with natural physics effects on your body just as love and hugs too.

Each chapter I have written is aimed to be easy and like a coffee chat with a friend who's been there, done that, and figured out how to make fitness less of a chore and more of a joy.

Whether you're here to tone up, gain energy, or just want to keep dancing like nobody's watching, this guide is your partner in crime (well, maybe more like your partner in plank). So, lace up your trainers, roll out that yoga mat, and let's show the world and ourselves that the best is yet to come.

Let's do this, one laugh and one lunge at a time!

As One Energy Together

Amanda xxx

I have designed this book to be able to pick it up at any chapter on any day to follow and get ideas on your fitness journey. I am all about nature, keeping programs simple and easy for you on your daily travels. The gym wasn't for me unless I was training for a race. In my experience, most women who pay and start with their New Year resolutions are very short-lived. A gym owner told me in Spain if everyone who signed up for a gym membership arrived on the same day they would never cope.

Always be a work in progress

— Emily Lillian

Most gym memberships are taken out early in the new year and when summer hits, everyone wants to be outside. The way I see it is everywhere you look is your free gym. Never lose the opportunity wherever you are to stretch or perform some easy exercises as I always have, I have gotten over people asking me what I am doing. I always say training for a 5km and they are satisfied that it is important to train for this.

10 Common Issues Senior Women Fear Over 60

In my book for you, I aim to address all your worries and fears about starting your fitness journey. For those of you restarting with some fitness experience (e.g., yoga, walking, or dancing) but lack consistency and are Interested in healthy aging, maintaining independence, or combating age-related challenges then this book is for you.

Some of you may have some prior experience with fitness (e.g., yoga, walking, or dancing) but lack consistency. Here are my top 10 issues:

1. **Fatigue** & Low Energy is a key issue.
2. **Struggling** to maintain stamina throughout the day.
3. **Joint Pain** or Stiffness.
4. **Difficulty moving** freely due to arthritis or general wear-and-tear.
5. **Body Image** Concerns.
6. **Feeling self-conscious** about aging bodies, sagging skin, or weight gain.
7. **Fear** of Injuries.
8. **Worry** about falling or getting hurt while exercising.
9. **Lack** of Motivation and stress
10. **Procrastinating** or feeling overwhelmed by starting a fitness journey.

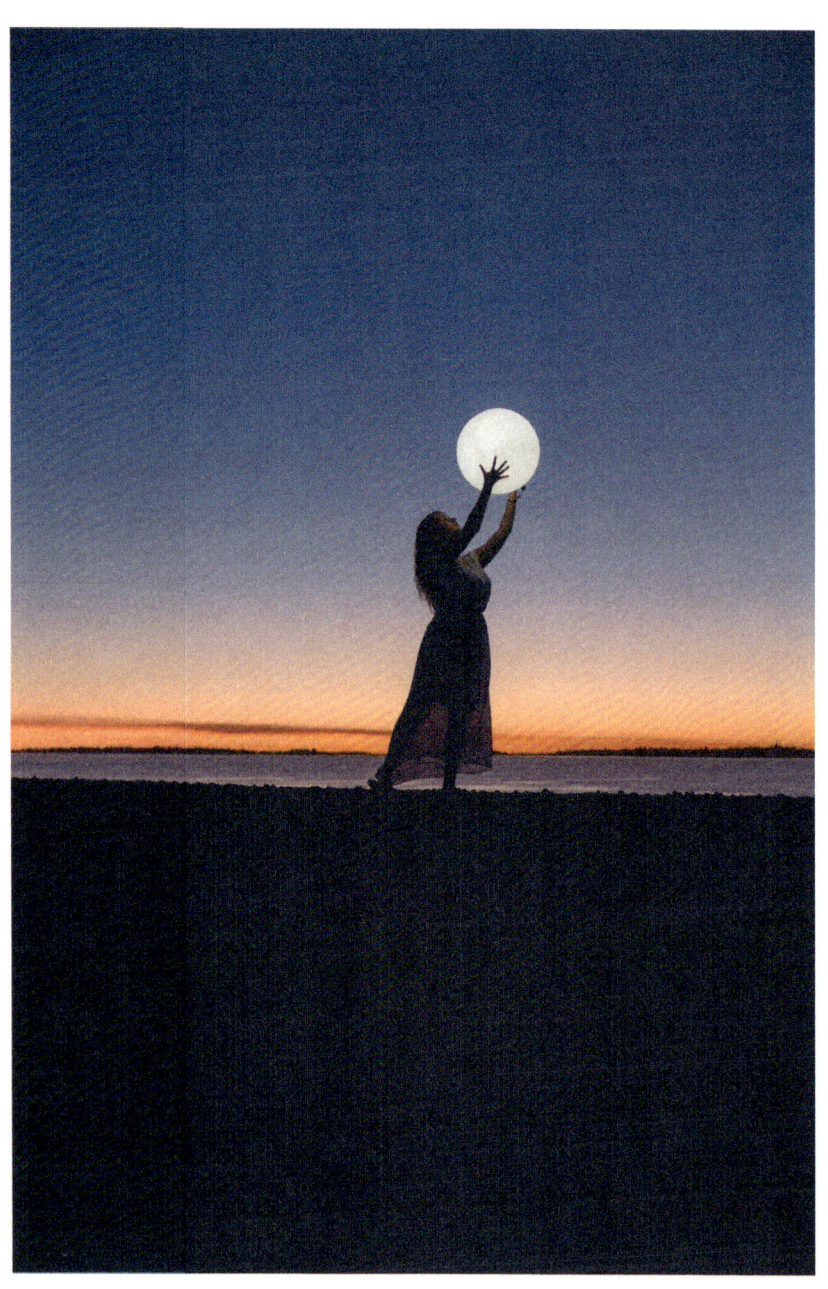

The World is Your Oyster

Age Is Just a Number, Darling!

Let's set the record straight. Being a Senior woman over 60 is fabulous. You will learn how to embrace your age with grace and confidence along with the funny side of life inside this book.

You've earned every laugh line, every silver strand, and the "Oh, I could tell you some stories" glance. Age isn't a limitation; it's a badge of honor. And when it comes to fitness, who says you can't teach an old dog or, as I prefer, a wise wolf a few new tricks?

"You are never too old to set another goal or to dream a new dream."
— **C.S. Lewis**

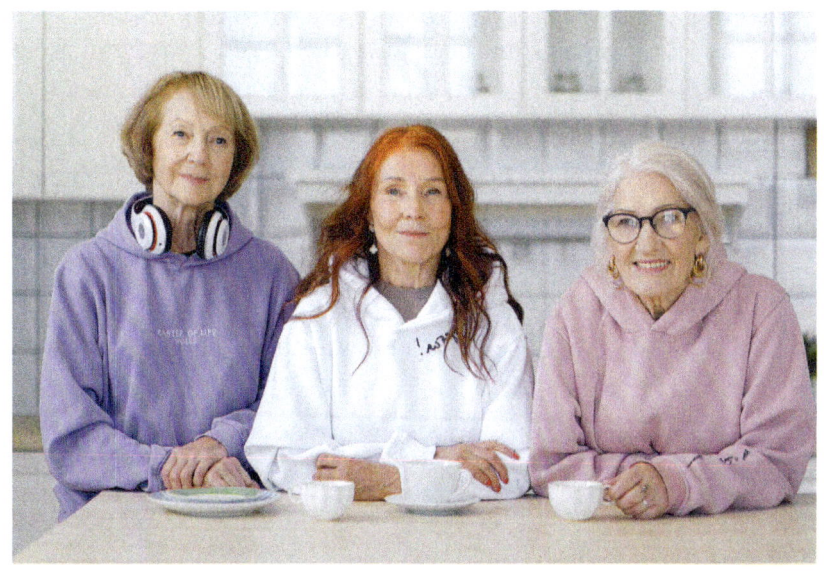

Fitness With Friends Old and New

"It's never too late to pursue your dreams and live life to the fullest".

"At 60+, finding your fitness groove is like finding your glasses, it takes some effort, but once you do, everything's clearer!"

Finding What Feels Right

Now, you've probably heard it all before:

"At your age, you should take it easy."

"Weights? Aren't those for younger people?"

"Just stick to walking, darling, you don't want to hurt yourself."

Let me tell you something. The next time someone says, "Take it easy," smile sweetly and respond, "Oh, I will…after my deadlifts." Strength, energy, and mobility aren't reserved for 20-year-olds. Your older self knows how to train smarter; it just needs a little TLC and a touch of humor.

My best compliment from a lady was when I said I was training for a marathon. She said when you get to my age it's too late, your knees and bones ache. I asked how old you were. She replied, 50! Fifty, I exclaimed. Do you know how old I am? No, she replied. Laughing, I said I was 60 and just moved into a new race category. My grandmother used to say you do not feel any different with age. I did wonder what age she decided to stop, the 30s, 40s, or 50s.

The oldest lady I welcomed as a guest was Anna from Denmark, who arrived with her daughter for two weeks at age 81. Anna was looking for a new start proving that there is always another challenge, another goal to plan since losing her husband of many years. Starting over at 81 can be very daunting. We quickly established she used to love hiking and was keen to see if she could start hiking again with a senior holiday group she wanted to join. With Anna, she needed confidence and leg strength, her mindset was strong. Proving age does not have to be a barrier.

The Valencia Marathon below was my first long road race challenge off the mountain trails at 58.

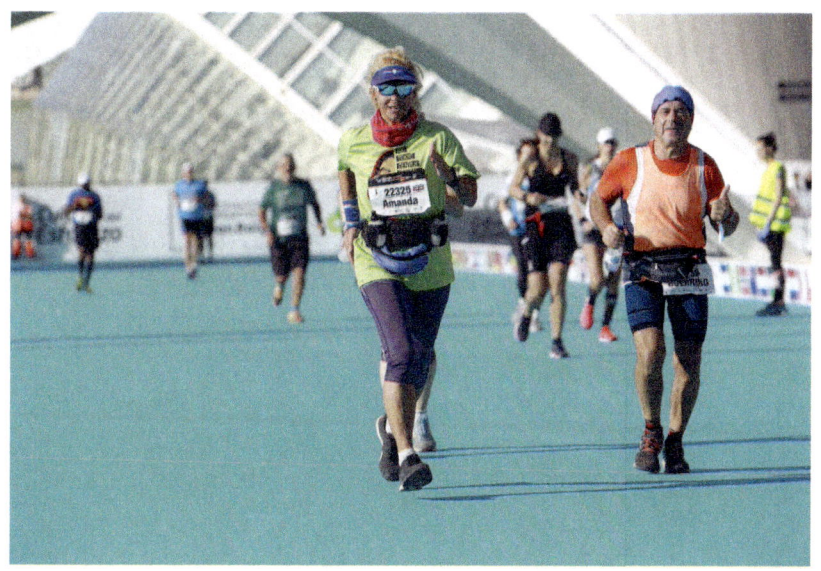

My First Marathon in 2019 in Valencia Spain

Now I understand. The mirror may have a different version of me, but without my reading glasses I pretend I do not need to see the years, therefore, yes I feel the same, in fact, I feel fitter and stronger now than in my 40s!

Picture this. You're striding into the gym or your living room, let's be honest with your water bottle in one hand and your **"I can do this"** attitude in the other. Someone whispers, "She's how old?" And you laugh to yourself, thinking, Watch and learn kiddo.

Fitness at 60+ isn't about six-pack abs or running marathons (unless you're into that). It's about keeping up with grandkids, dancing like nobody's watching, and feeling strong enough to carry the groceries without needing a nap afterward.

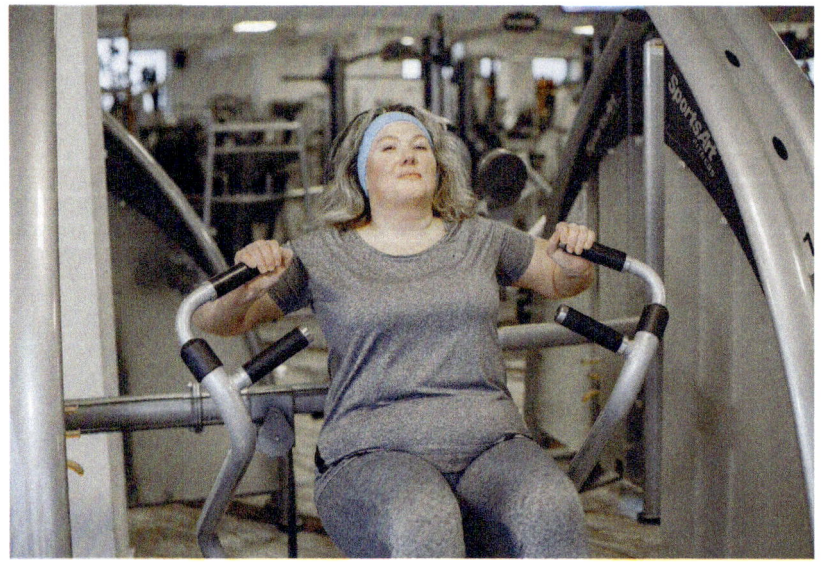

Go Easy to Start, always ask for a beginners program from the gym coach

Victory loves preparation. First and most important is to **plan your weekly sessions** and the day before or night at bedtime imagine yourself on your chosen session or walk where will you go? Take a mental journey and you will find the next day your session flows perfectly. Plan your day. Will you need a snack or extra water? What about your kit? Where can you shower and change? If not toilets and wipes or a small micro towel for a quick freshen up before that coffee or shopping. Plan a routine and have a goal to aim for. **Start your diary or journal from day 1 my top tip.**

Essential Requirements to Kickstart Your Fitness Program and Life Transformation

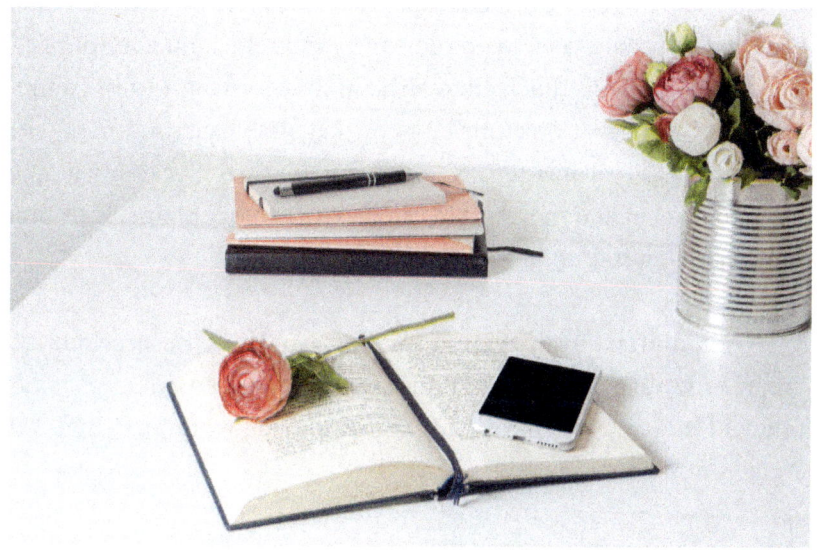

Journal and Plan Your Week from the Outset

Let's begin here:

Mindset Decision. Decide to prioritize your health and fitness. Set clear, achievable goals and commit to making this transformation for *you*.

Consult Your Medical Professional. Schedule a **health check-up** to discuss your plans, ensure you're ready to commence your activity and address any medical concerns or limitations. Continue to report along the way. Diet may be an issue consult with a nutritionist for training dietary advice **at the start.**

Invest in a Progress Journal. Track your journey! Record your daily progress, set goals, celebrate milestones, and reflect on your physical and mental growth. Block out dedicated time for your fitness routine and activities. Treat this time as a non-negotiable appointment with yourself to ensure consistency. You inform others, if it's easier you have an appointment and they won't even dare to ask where. It is your time to block out, just for you.

Visit a Podiatrist or Specialist for Gait Analysis. Ensure your feet are in good shape and invest in the right footwear based on your gait to avoid injuries and maximize comfort during workouts. Invest in Walker foot plasters.

Gear Up. Check your wardrobe for fitness-appropriate clothing. Invest in comfortable, moisture-wicking activewear and supportive undergarments designed for mature women.

Tech Check. Consider purchasing a fitness tracker, app, or simple pedometer to monitor your activity, heart rate, and progress. A smartwatch or step counter can also be a great motivational tool.

Build a Supportive Environment. Create a space for home workouts, whether it's yoga, stretching, or light resistance training. Add smaller items like resistance bands, dumbbells, or yoga mats to your starter kit.

Plan Your Meals and Hydration. Set up a simple, nutritious meal plan. Stock your kitchen with wholesome foods and a good reusable water bottle to stay hydrated throughout the day.

Schedule Time for Recovery and Rest. Build recovery days into your routine. Rest is just as important as exercise for achieving long-term success. Include stretches, mindfulness practices, or even a relaxing nap.

Find Your Community. Join a class, group, or online community of like-minded women who share your goals. Having a support network is key to staying motivated. Your journey with others makes the process more enjoyable and helps keep you on track.

Aging's Perks. Let's not forget the unique benefits of this age:

No one expects you to be on Instagram showing off your squat form (but you really could).

You've mastered the art of saying "no" to things that don't serve you like diets named after colors.

You get to roll your eyes at fitness trends that come and go faster than a Zumba class warm-up.

A Call to Action ladies. So, what are you waiting for? Join me as we begin your journey. Lace up your trainers, grab a light dumbbell, and begin by taking a deep breath and moving those arms. You're not too old, weak, or too late to start. You're exactly where you're supposed to be: ready for a fresh start with a side of sass.

Remember, darling, you're 60+ fabulous, and fearless. Let's show the world what that looks like. If you were a Masters Athletics athlete you would be called a Senior Vet at 35! A definite medal of honor.

The Power of Positivity in Fitness One of the greatest things about being a senior woman over 60 is having the **wisdom** to know that perfection isn't the **goal** progress is. Your fitness **journey** isn't about running marathons (unless you want to) or becoming the world's next yoga guru. It's about feeling **strong**, capable, and **confident** in your skin.

Let's start with a few truths:

1. You don't need to spend hours in the gym. Consistency matters more than duration.

2. Fitness doesn't have to hurt to be effective. If it hurts, you're either doing it wrong or doing too much.

3. It's okay to laugh at yourself especially when you're trying something new. (Remember the first time you used resistance bands and they turned into a slingshot? No? Just me?)

This reminds me of my first time holding resistance bands, let me share a quick tale. My first attempt at using one was at home, without instructions. I hooked it onto my doorknob, tugged at it, and bam! it snapped back like a rubber band on steroids. I spent the next hour icing my dignity (and my forehead). Lesson learned: read the instructions and start slow!

These moments aren't failures; they're badges of honor. Each wobble in yoga or wrong step in Zumba is proof that you're showing up and trying. Zumba, I never could get all the steps and always ended up freestyling, but having a good time and a sweat to finish. Laugh and enjoy.

Take it from Sharon, who joined her first Pilates class with me in Spain and accidentally did half the workout facing the wrong direction; easily done, as the teacher moved around demonstrating for all to see. Mirroring left and right can be a challenge when you have no idea what's going on the first week. Go with the flow. Sharon's instructor, who had not said a word until the end of the class, asked kindly if she'd enjoyed her 'customized session. They laughed so hard, she signed up for the next class immediately.

Fitness is about showing up, having fun, and not taking yourself too seriously.

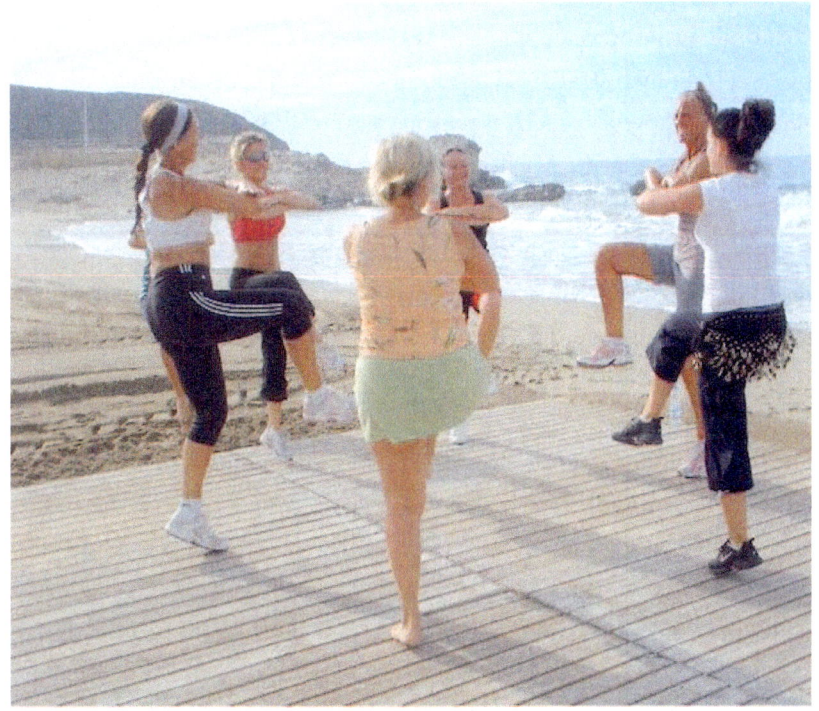

Shirley teaching her first-ever Zumba class, it was a giggle with the girls

Fitness isn't one-size-fits-all. Some women love the camaraderie of a group class, while others prefer the quiet solitude of a morning walk. The key is to experiment and find what fits you.

Here are 2 easy ideas to get you started:

Walking, Whether it's in a park, around your neighborhood, or on a treadmill, walking is an excellent way to get your heart rate up without putting too much strain on your joints. I find it best even as a runner. A sense of purpose or practical reason to go walking is easy when there's a goal such as posting a letter or buying some groceries or veggies. Or simply a cheeky coffee at your favorite coffee house either half time on your walk or the end as a treat, reward yourself for doing so.

Not having a car for one year, that was easy. I would plan my daily trips to the shops via the woods or the park to get some extra time on my feet.

Dancing, Modern jive, ballroom, or just grooving in your living room dancing is cardio disguised as fun. If you are single reading this at any age but in your 60s Modern Jive or ballroom or Salsa is a wonderful way to meet new friends and who knows maybe Cupid makes a strike just when you least expect it. Like-minded folks are to be found here too.

If you are in a relationship, go together and rekindle your disco days with your partner. Soon keeping fit and healthy will be the by-product of your fun nights out. Getting fit together will never be a chore doing something you love, that's the secret to life at any age.

These classes are held in every village, town, and city to be found nearly every evening of the week. This also includes many special 'Freestyle' events where you can put your new cool moves into practice. These evening classes and events can be researched online. There are many weekends and or 7-day holidays to be booked for even more fun fitness breaks.

Claire shared with me her first trip to a new dance fitness class, "I tried Zumba for the first time, and by the second song, I was wildly flapping my arms like a confused flamingo. But when I looked around, I realized everyone else was too! Now, I'm addicted."

What Fitness Gear Do I Need?

Buy a couple of backpacks in two sizes small and large with one for pure walking days to fit a

- A lightweight water bottle
- Emergency contact and any medical details on a waterproof card
- Tissues for all emergencies such as a call of nature! Keep waterproof
- Mobile and glasses (if needed) in a waterproof pouch
- Cotton buff to protect your neck in hot and cold weather
- Two plastic bags for any extra shopping, wet gear, foraging, or heavy rain to keep everything dry in your pack.
- A Small absorbent microfiber towel is perfect for drying your feet after a dip in the stream. You can purchase one online or from a running or walking shop.
- Sunglasses both for the sun, wind or even blasting rain from the fact
- Sun Hat with peak fends off rain and will keep the sun and rain off whilst warm
- Compact umbrella. The backpack should just hold these items and leave enough room for any smaller items you may wish to pack a healthy cereal bar
- Quality running shoes and walking shoes

- Leggings breathable sports tops and sports bra.

The large backpack is used for days out on the hills to carry your lunch and camera or for shopping trips filled with groceries. When using the bigger pack, take the contents from the smaller pack or simply keep extras from the above list. My large backpack is a walker's pack. I chose it because it has a special full rain cover built into a zipped area at the bottom for unexpected rainfall days.

Purchases can be made online or Ebay or social media, even quality options from charity shops for the budget and also supporting your favorite charity whilst buying. I have managed to buy all manner of fitness, walking, and running gear, and backpacks over the years.

I know what you are thinking. What next? Hey, it's a gym-free day. An all-in-one free distracted workout. A walk in nature with a trip to the local shops or weekly market or perhaps a coffee then load up with essential shopping just think load weight training. Strengthen those legs. Soon your ratio to fitness and weight will keep up with any Himalayan Sherpa traversing Everest without any effort!

Inspiring Stories

Meet Jenny, my mother who was 73 years old, recently widowed, and starting a single life again, she discovered modern jive dancing at her local community center after we had initially brainstormed with her. We talked about all her hobbies and things she would love to try now single and free to decide. We made a huge random list, but a clear pattern began to emerge such as walking, yoga, nature, and dancing. I Googled all the clubs and walking groups near her that offered beginners' classes and walkers. Soon my mother was taking her first Modern Jive class where most women were single and all worried about being by themselves too.

My mother; forever the social butterfly, made new friends easily with other ladies also single who enjoyed walking, and who shared the same gardening interests. She said to me after her evening class "At first, I thought I'd embarrass myself," she said. "But after a few classes, I realized everyone was stepping on each other's toes—literally. Being single was daunting but I was made to feel super welcome. I even decided to treat myself to a pair of dancing shoes, imagine at my age. Now, it's my favorite activity, and I've even joined a group that travels for competitions!"

Take Alice, a 67-year-old who decided to try hiking. She started with a small hill near her home and now tackles trails that would make her 40-year-old self very envious. "It's not about the distance," Alice insists. "It's about the journey and the snacks you pack."

These senior women proved that it's never too late to start something new when they joined one of my retreats in Spain.

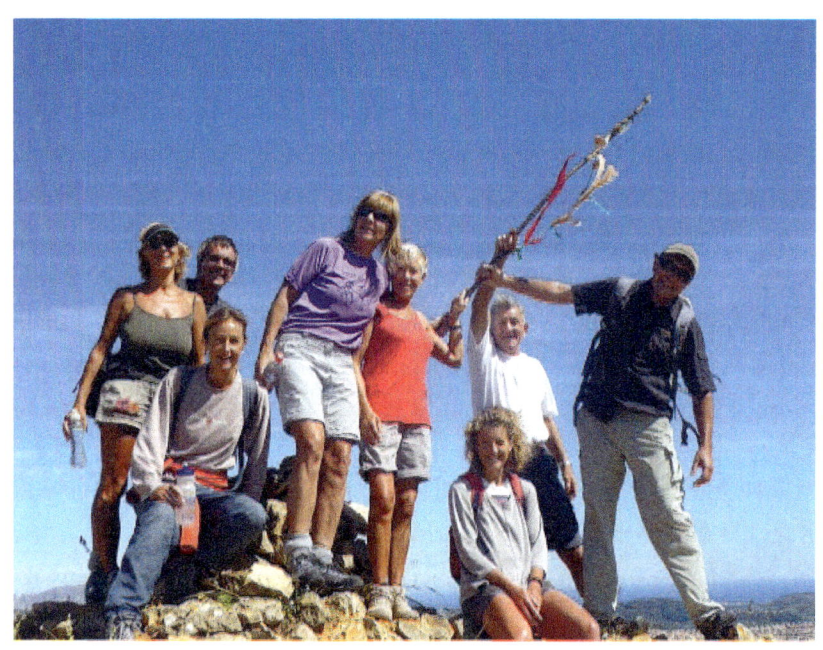

Reaching The Summit is The Best Feeling Ever

Your Weekly 5-Point Challenge Checklist

To help you stay motivated, here's a simple weekly challenge checklist. The goal is to tick off each item by the end of the week, giving you a sense of accomplishment and keeping your routine fresh.

Try a new activity. Challenge yourself to step out of your comfort zone. Maybe it's a Zumba class, a Tai chi session, or an aqua aerobics workout. If you're feeling adventurous, sign up for a free class at your local community center or gym.

"Change your thoughts and you change your world."
— **Norman Vincent Peale**

How It Helps. Keep fitness exciting and prevent boredom. Build confidence in your ability to adapt and learn. Every week vary what you do.

Tips for Success. Bringing a friend it's less intimidating and way more fun. Don't worry about "getting it right." The goal is to enjoy yourself.

When I was living in Spain, belly dancing classes were very popular. My friend Kate decided to join a belly dancing class for fun. Her first class she told me was hilarious, "I spent half the time tangled in my scarf and the other half trying to control my giggles. But by the end, I had a newfound respect for my hips and the instructor!"

Walk 5,000 Steps a Day (or More) or no less: Walking is one of the simplest ways to stay active, and it's easy to build into your day. Stroll around the block, explore a nearby trail, or walk laps at the mall if the weather isn't cooperating.

How It Helps. Boosts cardiovascular health and improves mood. Strengthens your legs and enhances endurance.
 Tips for Success. Use a fitness tracker or phone app to count your steps. Break it into smaller chunks if 5,000 steps feel overwhelming at first. Make sure your activity is never less than 60 minutes.
 Always think time on feet may feel less stressful for you than steps

and if you do not own or want to own a step-o- meter then go for time, which is what I do.

In Spain, whilst I was living there, the shopping mall speed walking was very popular not because it was cold but the long months of intense heat. The ladies could drive in their air-con cars to the underground cool car park and start their hour of speed walking before having lunch there in the airy cool shopping mall. Perfect ingenious form of free fitness to suit your lifestyle. Think out of the box to make your daily life fitness pure fun with no gym effort. The gym I know doesn't suit everyone.

One Spanish lady told me as I was intrigued to see these rather fit older ladies whizzing past me at top speed as I sat enjoying my coffee shed, found the perfect fitness plan, and made new like-minded friends too. She had discovered the joys of mall walking when she unintentionally joined a group of seniors speed-walking. "I was just trying to window-shop, but I ended up in a high-speed race to the food court!" I loved her story of how she started.

Strength Train Twice A Week. Lifting weights or using resistance bands isn't about "bulking up." It's about keeping your muscles and bones strong, which is especially important as we age.

How It Helps. Reduces the risk of osteoporosis. Enhances functional strength for everyday tasks like lifting groceries.
  Tips for Success. Start light—2-5 lbs is perfect for beginners. Focus on form rather than how much weight you're lifting.
  Lifting weights or using resistance bands isn't about "bulking up." It's about keeping your muscles and bones strong, which is especially important as we age.

Note to yourself always carry a healthy cereal bar.

Beth learned the hard way not to skip breakfast before strength training. "Halfway through, I got so lightheaded, that I started lifting imaginary weights to keep up with the group. Nobody noticed—except the trainer, who handed me a granola bar!"

Stretch Every Day. Flexibility is key to staying agile and preventing injury. Spend just 5-10 minutes a day stretching your major muscle groups. Bonus points if you do it while watching TV or listening to music. I always prefer to do standing stretches in the shower. It's invigorating, relaxing, and a safe undisturbed place of 'Me Time'.

How It Helps: Improves range of motion. Relieves tension and reduces stiffness.

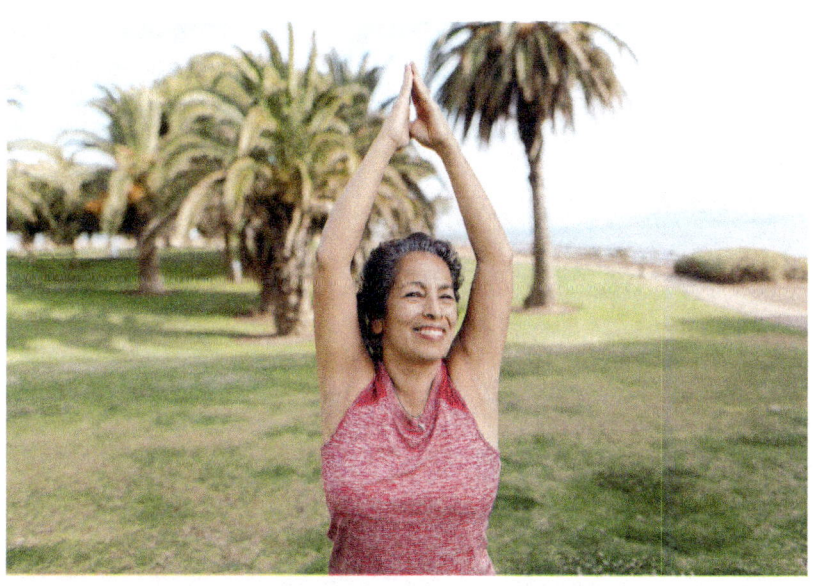

Make daily stretching a part of "The New You"

Tips for Success: Include neck, shoulder, and lower back stretch. Don't bounce—stretch gently and hold for 15-30 seconds. Gently close your eyes and breathe letting it all go relax. Turn your mind to that specific muscle you are stretching, imagine it stretching and releasing softly. This is when your yoga moves will kick in here making it much easier.

During one stretch session, I was helping my friend Jane, when her husband Steve walked in, took one look at her attempt to touch her toes, and said, "Are you trying to find your lost keys?" whoops.

"The five S's of Sports training are: stamina, speed, strength, skill, and spirit; but the greatest of these is spirit" ~ **Ken Doherty** Snooker Player

Spirit means the will to succeed to believe, you set your sights to achieve.

Schedule a "Fun Day". Fitness isn't all about structure. Once a week, do something active that feels like pure fun. Go dancing, play with your grandkids, garden, or enjoy a bike ride. The goal is to move your body and forget that you're "exercising."

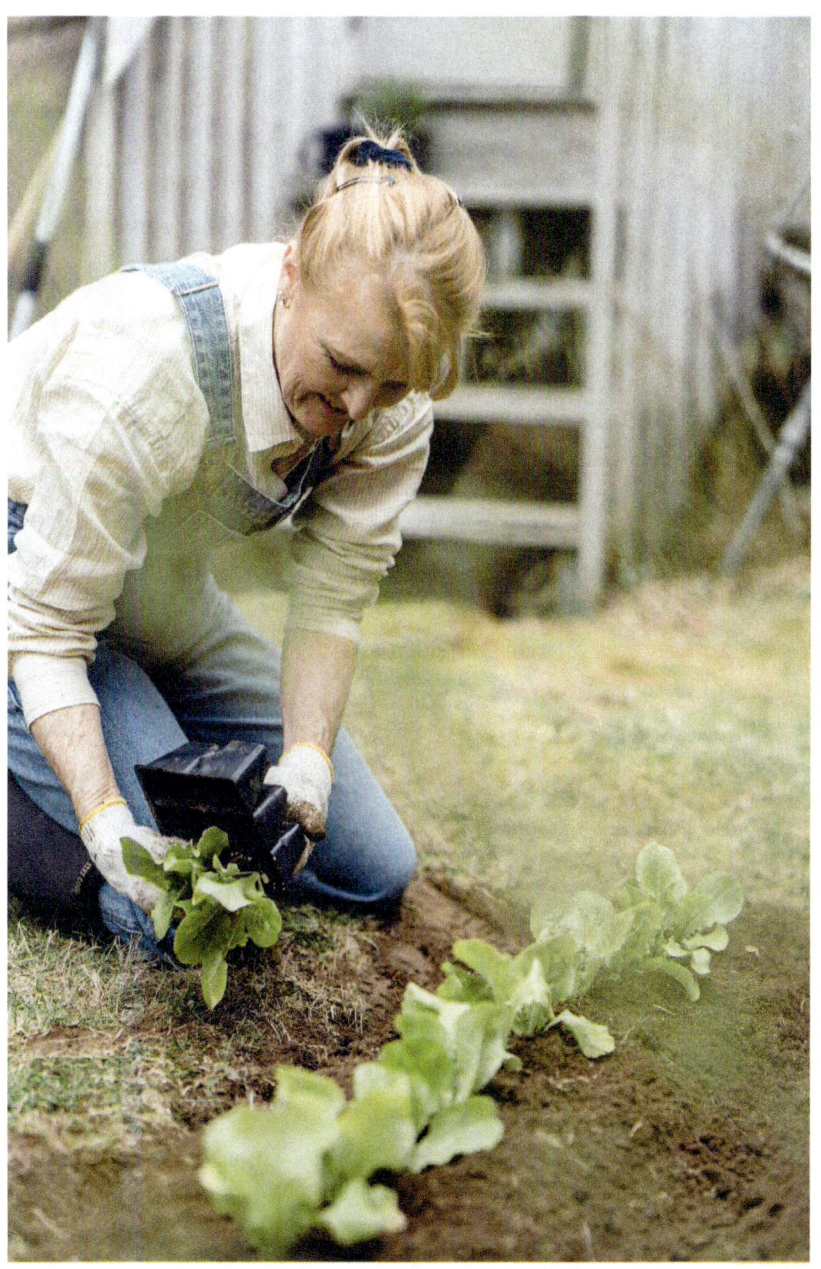

Gardening guaranteed to relax and even sweat

How It Helps. Reinforces the idea that fitness can be enjoyable. Keep yourself motivated by mixing up your activities.

Tips for Success. Pick something that makes you smile just thinking about it. Invite others to join—laughter is the best workout buddy.

When Pat joined her grandson for a game of backyard tag, she found herself outsmarted at every turn. "He has endless energy, but I have a strategy. I bribed him with cookies to let me win!" It has to be done.

My husband is the champion of this strategy. He loves to win at any age with his forever competitive mind, even at 66 he can still outsprint most thirty-somethings as a UK GB Masters triple gold medallist in 2019. It took two years of dedicated training once he decided to set his goals to achieve his target. Not that you would want to be a master, just to demonstrate what is possible in a short time. You can do anything you want.

"Set realistic goals, keep re-evaluating, and be consistent"
   ~ **Venus Williams**

Mindset Matters

Your mindset is your most powerful tool. Replace "I can't" with "I'm learning," and celebrate every small victory. Remember, showing up is the hardest part—and you're already a pro.

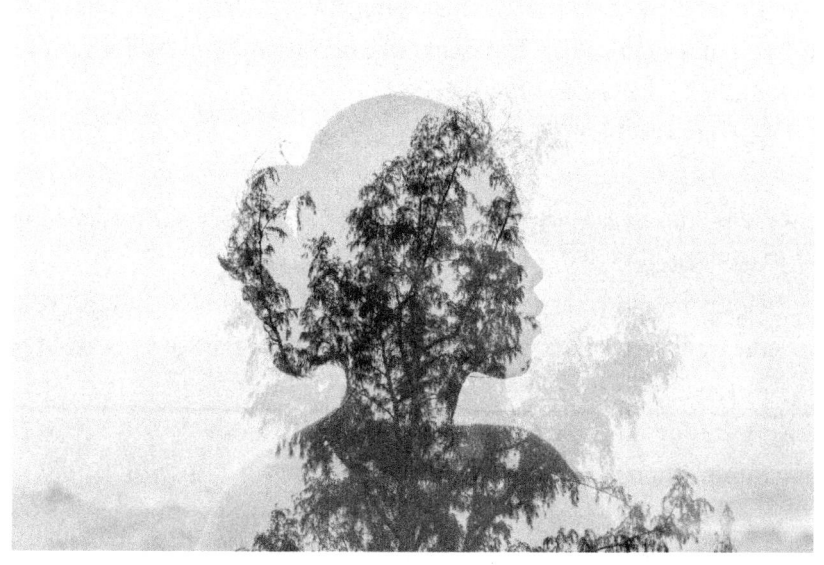

Your energy goes where your mind flows, listen to your inner talk

Hilarious Hiccups Are Part of the Fun. Fitness bloopers are a rite of passage. Whether it's tripping over your yoga mat or mistaking your water bottle for your grandchild's sippy cup, these moments remind us not to take life too seriously.

Journaling Your Journey

Consider keeping a fitness journal to track your progress. Write down what you tried, what you loved, and even what made you laugh. It's not about recording numbers—it's about reflecting on how you feel.

My next project is to write an accompanying journal to fit this book for you to write in daily. It is one of the best tools I created for my use over the years based on my experience.

Each day it will consist of:

- Your chosen activity? I always record my distance run/walked my GPS watch
- How long do you spend doing it? Remember time on your feet is the most important. Whatever you can achieve in your 60 minutes or longer for walks daily
- Your food intake, what did each meal consist of?
- Super important how you felt marks out of ten with 10 being fabulous and under 5 not so. Question: why? illness etc
- The weather record?
- Menopausal symptoms?
- Your rest/family days strike out on your weekly calendar.

By the end of each week and month, you will very quickly begin to see patterns of fabulous few cyclical days or opposite or lack of sleep from late nights, etc. This will keep you on the right track. Set your goals and targets for the month, and the year as soon as you start. It may be a fitness/walking holiday, family with the grandkids, or a race or special event.

Conclusion Final Words of Encouragement

Your fitness groove is uniquely yours. It doesn't matter what anyone else is doing or what worked for them. What matters is finding something that brings you joy and makes you feel alive.

Remember you will only ever regret the days when you didn't go out for your exercise. No matter what fitness you do, you will always feel great and mentally be so glad you did.

So, go ahead—put on those trainers, pick an activity, and start moving. Remember, darling, age is just a number, and you're about to prove it!

Stretching the Truth (and Your Hamstrings)

Understanding your body's signals is vital for maintaining a sustainable fitness routine at any age, but especially at 60 and beyond. Learning to listen to aches, energy levels, and recovery times is the difference between thriving and overdoing it. However, this chapter isn't just about serious advice because what's life without a little laughter?

Sometimes, our bodies send signals that we misinterpret (or hilariously ignore), and those moments are worth cherishing too.

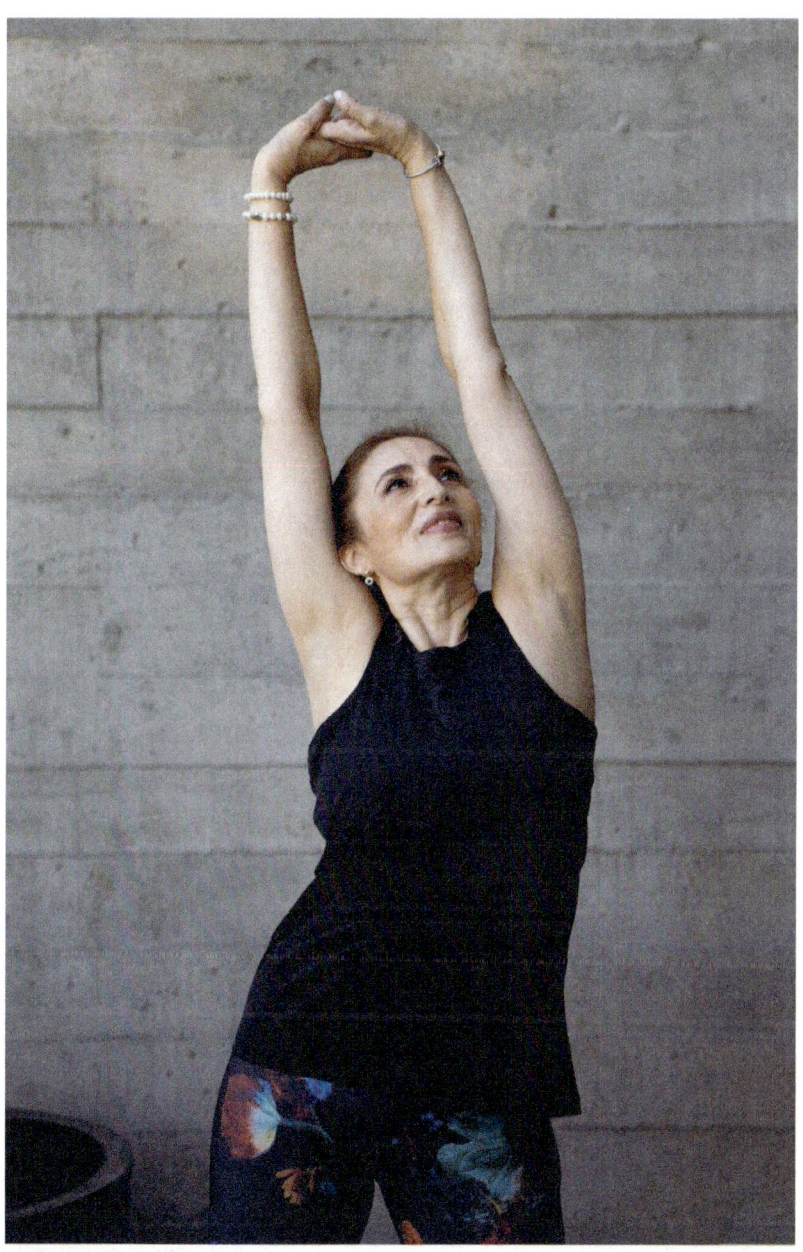

You can stretch anywhere at any time. The morning shower is my favorite place

Listen to Your Body-And Laugh While You Do. Understanding your body's signals is vital for maintaining a sustainable fitness routine at any age, but especially at 60 and beyond. Learning to listen to aches, energy levels, and recovery times is the difference between thriving and overdoing it.

However, this chapter isn't just about serious advice because what's life without a little laughter? Sometimes, our bodies send signals that we misinterpret (or hilariously ignore), and those moments are worth cherishing too.

Why Flexibility is the Key

Why Stretching Matters. More So over 60 or Whatever your age to be honest avoiding injuries is super important every single day during your day get into the stretching habit.

As we age, our muscles naturally lose some elasticity. Stretching keeps them supple, reduces stiffness, and improves range of motion. Plus, it just feels fantastic like giving your body a well-deserved hug.

Benefits of Stretching over 60

Reduces the risk of injury by loosening tight muscles.

- Improves posture, which makes you look taller (and who doesn't want that?).
- Helps alleviate aches and pains, especially in the lower back and joints.
- Enhances circulation for better energy.
- Gives you an excuse to pause during the day and take a deep breath.

Fun Task. Try a simple hamstring stretch during your favorite TV show's commercial break. It's multitasking at its finest, you'll feel productive while catching up on the latest drama (both on-screen and in your body).

We have all had to start somewhere and in my experience personally and for those I have helped to start their fitness journeys from zero is always too much too soon. Typically after two weeks, many give up, with sore aching muscles and feeling no immediate benefits or appearing to progress after aiming for a fast-track enthusiastic start.

Remember this is aimed to be a fun lifestyle change for the rest of your life not just 6 or 12 weeks. For many a diet or fitness plan to run a 5 km or half marathon for charity is simply a goal to be had which post-event becomes a massive sense of loss after the plan ends.

This is the first myth to dispel it's for life. I will share the fitness secrets and tips that have consistently worked for me. I have perfected and tested various approaches that I believe help women, including myself, create a natural lifestyle that is easy to maintain forever—far beyond a 12-week program followed by years of returning to old habits. I have gained in-depth knowledge to help you achieve your fitness. We will do it together here.

When one of my ladies Sue decided to "listen to her body" by skipping any leg strengthening exercises…for five years. "My legs didn't have much to say," she joked. When she finally added squats to her routine, her body made up for the silence with days of protests she could feel every time she sat down. There are much easier ways to escape the gym if it isn't for you.

Warming Up with Wit. "Warming up isn't optional unless you enjoy moving like a rusty tin man."

Ah, stretching the quiet hero of fitness. It's the part most of us skip because, honestly, who has time for all that bending and twisting? But let's face it: Without stretching, your muscles are about as cooperative as a toddler who missed naptime. Bend, Don't Break.

Flexibility is often overlooked in fitness routines, but it's the secret sauce to aging gracefully. Stretching isn't just about limbering up; it's about staying mobile, improving posture, and, most importantly, being able to tie your shoes without a crane. Over 60, stretching isn't optional, it's essential.

When you think about stretching, forget the intimidating images of young yogis twisting into pretzels. Flexibility at this stage is about comfort, longevity, and feeling good in your body. And let's face it: some stretches might look more like you're reaching for the cookies on the top shelf than auditioning for Cirque du Soleil and that's perfectly okay.

Sarah during her first yoga class, got into downward dog and immediately heard a loud pop. Panicked, she froze and whispered, "Was that my hip or my mat?" The instructor assured her it was the mat, but Sarah muttered, "Thank goodness. I was ready to call emergency services!"

The Morning Stretch Saga. Picture this: It's 7 a.m. You stretch your arms over your head, hear three pops, and think, Was that my back or my furniture? Fear not! That's just your body reminding you it's awake. Stretching isn't about perfection, it's about gently waking up those muscles and saying, "Hey, we've got a great day ahead."

Three Fun Stretches That Won't Break You (Or Your Furniture)

The Standing Sway: Stand tall, reach for the sky, and sway side to side like a graceful tree. Bonus points if you don't knock over a lamp.

Toe-Touch Tango: Bend down slowly to touch your toes—or your knees, or your shins, because we're all friends here.

Seated Twist: Sit on a chair, twist to one side, and imagine you're casually eavesdropping on your neighbor's juicy gossip.

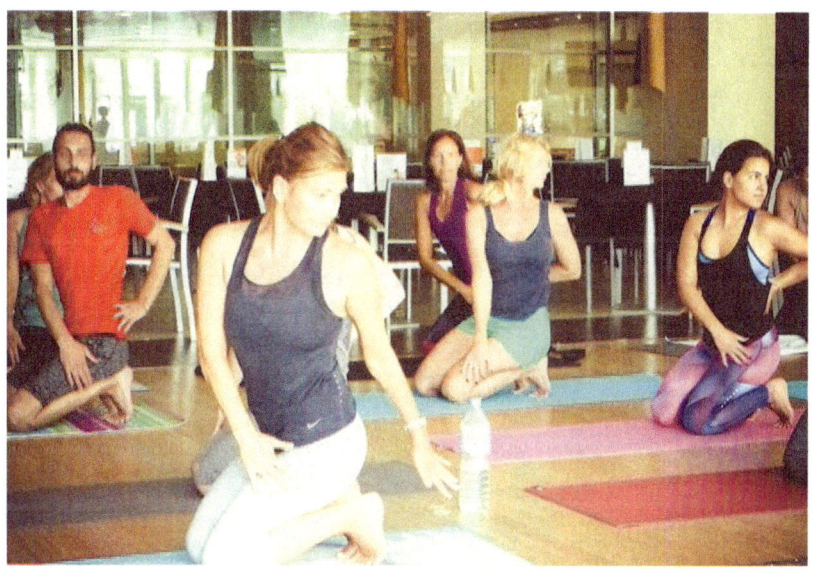

A yoga twist can be on the Floor or seated you choose

The Joy of Warming Up—Because Nobody Wants to Pull a Hamstring

Warming up before a workout isn't just a suggestion; it's a non-negotiable. Skipping it is like diving into a pool without testing the water you're setting yourself up for a shock. But don't worry, warming up doesn't have to be boring. It can be downright hilarious if you let it.

The Science of Warming Up. A proper warm-up gets your blood flowing, loosens your joints, and preps your muscles for action. Think of it as a polite wake-up call for your body, saying, "Hey, we're about to do something here. Time to shake off the cobwebs!"

Stretching for Every Occasion. Stretching doesn't have to be confined to workout sessions. Incorporate it into your daily life for maximum benefits:

Morning Stretch. Start your day with a simple reach for the sky stretch. Bonus: you'll look like a victorious superhero. Stretch up to those shelves at the supermarket or bend down a few times pretending to get something from the bottom shelf.

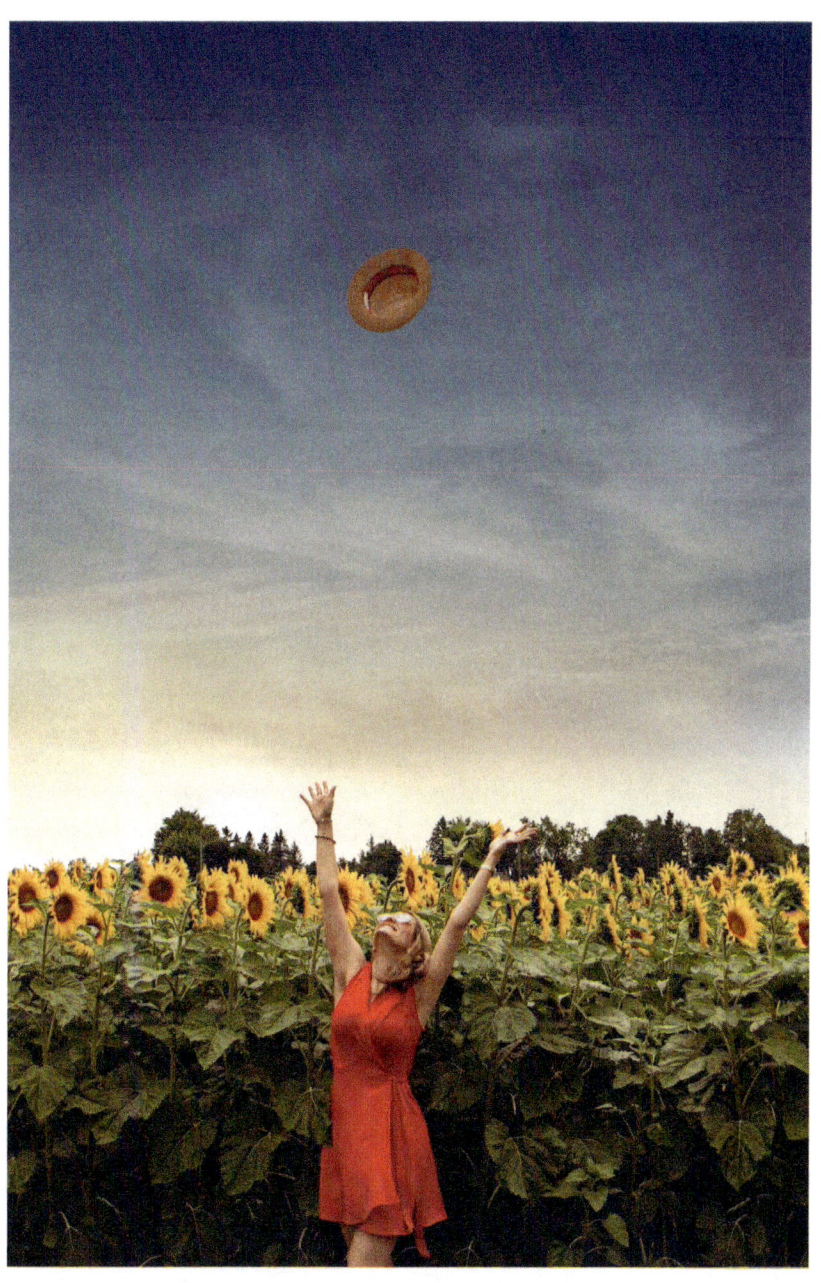

Reach for the sky anywhere anytime

Midday Stretch. Combat desk slump by rolling your shoulders and doing a seated spinal twist. Whilst out getting creative, I have always learned to never waste an opportunity throughout your day to stretch. Stretch anywhere on railings, park benches, or in the public toilets in a cubicle if necessary!

Evening Stretch. A Child's pose with a gentle forward fold before bed helps relax your body and mind.

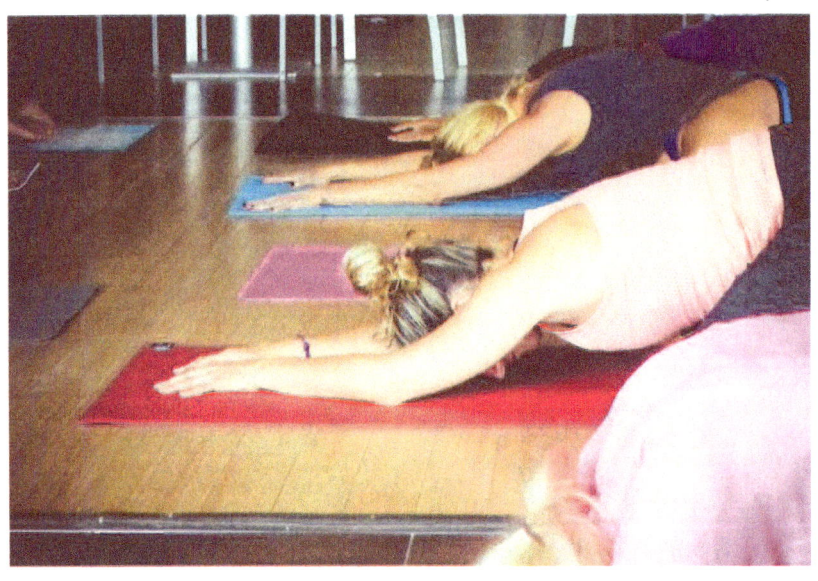

A yoga restorative pose called The Child's Pose

Fun Task. Create a "Stretching Bingo" card with moves like a hamstring stretch, shoulder roll, or child's pose. Cross them off as you go and reward yourself when you complete a row (perhaps with chocolate?).

Stretch anywhere on railings, park benches, or in the public toilets in a cubicle if necessary!

My neighbor Helen, 70, began incorporating stretches into her gardening routine. "I call it 'yoga with weeds,'" she says. "Not only does it make pulling weeds easier, but I've also noticed my knees don't complain as much anymore!"

But let's face it, warming up can feel awkward. There's nothing quite like swinging your arms in a circle and wondering if you're channeling a windmill or attempting a slow-motion karate chop.

The "Forgot My Balance" Stretch. You're standing on one leg, pulling your other foot back to stretch your quad, feeling proud until you topple over like a tree in slow motion. It's fine; trees are majestic, and so are you. I suggest you always look for a railing or a tree for this one.

The Surprise Snap. Ever done a toe touch and heard a crack that makes you wonder if you've just dislocated something? Don't worry; it's probably just your joints letting out a groan of disapproval for skipping this step last week.

The Mirror Mishap. If you've ever done a warm-up in front of a mirror, you know the struggle. You start with good intentions, but halfway through, you're distracted by your funny expressions or a stray hair doing its workout.

The "Forgot My Keys" Jog. Jog on the same on the spot, while pretending to look for your keys. Bonus points for muttering, "I just had them a second ago!"

The Coffee Reach. Stand tall and stretch as if reaching for a coffee mug on the top shelf. Hold that stretch—it's the caffeine you need to fuel your day!

The Air Guitar Solo. Strum your invisible guitar while rocking out to your favorite tune. Not only will your arms get a good stretch, but you'll also feel like a rock star.

The "Shoo the Cat" Sidestep. Shuffle to the side as if gently nudging a curious cat out of your workout space. Don't forget to throw in an exaggerated arm wave for flair.

Why Warming Up is Better Over 60

At this age, warming up becomes a necessity and a source of comedy gold. You've got life experience on your side, which means you're less embarrassed about the funny noises your body makes during a warm-up. Groaning? Cracking? That's just the soundtrack of a body that's been around the block—and it's still raring to go. No one will pay you any attention wearing your fitness gear, you will feel the part.

Stretching slowly can also aid sleep faster as it is very relaxing, make it a habit you will feel great.

Plus plenty tends to happen sitting or lying down on your mat!

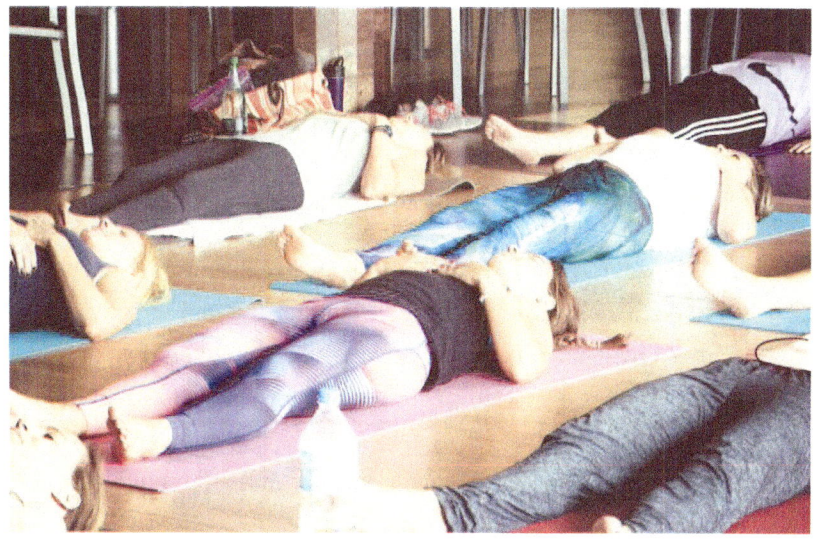

The relaxation pose of the class is called Shavasana or the Corpse Pose

Warming Up with a Partner. Double the Fun. Grab a friend or partner and make warming up a social event.

The Handshake Stretch. Greet each other with an exaggerated handshake, then stretch out those arm muscles.

The Salsa Shimmy. Loosen your shoulders with a quick shimmy. If it turns into a mini dance-off, all the better!

The Laughing Lunge. Try lunging side by side while telling your favorite jokes. Warning: sudden bursts of laughter may disrupt your balance.

Finding joy in flexibility; yes, there is. Warming up and stretching isn't just a physical activity; it's a mental one, too. It forces you to slow down and be present, something we all need in this fast-paced world.

As you gently close your eyes and flow into your chosen routine of muscle stretches, take your mind's eye to that muscle and feel it relaxing and surrendering to you as you breathe into it. Soon you will begin to flow, move to where you need the attention most, and just breathe and let it all out. Then your muscles will love you and give in slowly.

Top 5 Ways to Make Stretching Fun

- **Add Music.** Create a playlist of your favorite relaxing tunes.
- **Do It With Friends.** Turn stretching into a social activity.
- **Stretch Outdoors.** Fresh air makes everything better.
- **Laugh at Yourself:** Embrace the moments when you wobble or lose balance.
- **Reward Progress:** Celebrate when you can finally touch your toes (or even your knees).
- Book a Yin Yoga evening class. Yin is a gentle form of yoga and very relaxing

When Sally invited her best friend to a stretching session in the park, they ended up giggling uncontrollably while trying to balance in a tree pose. "We were more like wobbling saplings," she quips, "but we had a blast!"

"Flexibility is the key to stability."
— **John Wooden**

3 Common Stretching Mistakes (and How to Avoid Them)

Stretching may look simple, but it's easy to get it wrong. Here's how to avoid turning your morning stretch into an unintentional comedy routine.

Mistake #1: Bouncing While Stretching. It's tempting to bob up and down, but this can strain your muscles. Instead, hold each stretch steady for 20–30 seconds.

Mistake #2: Skipping the Warm-Up. Stretching cold muscles is like trying to unfold a frozen garden hose. Always do light activity first to warm up.

Mistake #3: Comparing Yourself to Others. Your flexibility journey is uniquely yours. It's not a competition—unless you're competing with your cat, in which case, good luck.

"Rather than focusing on the obstacle in your path, focus on the bridge over the obstacle." – **Mary Lou Retton.**

Henriette at 71 my inspirational running buddy the 'Stretch Queen', post race with cheila her dog on a park bench working those hamstrings out.

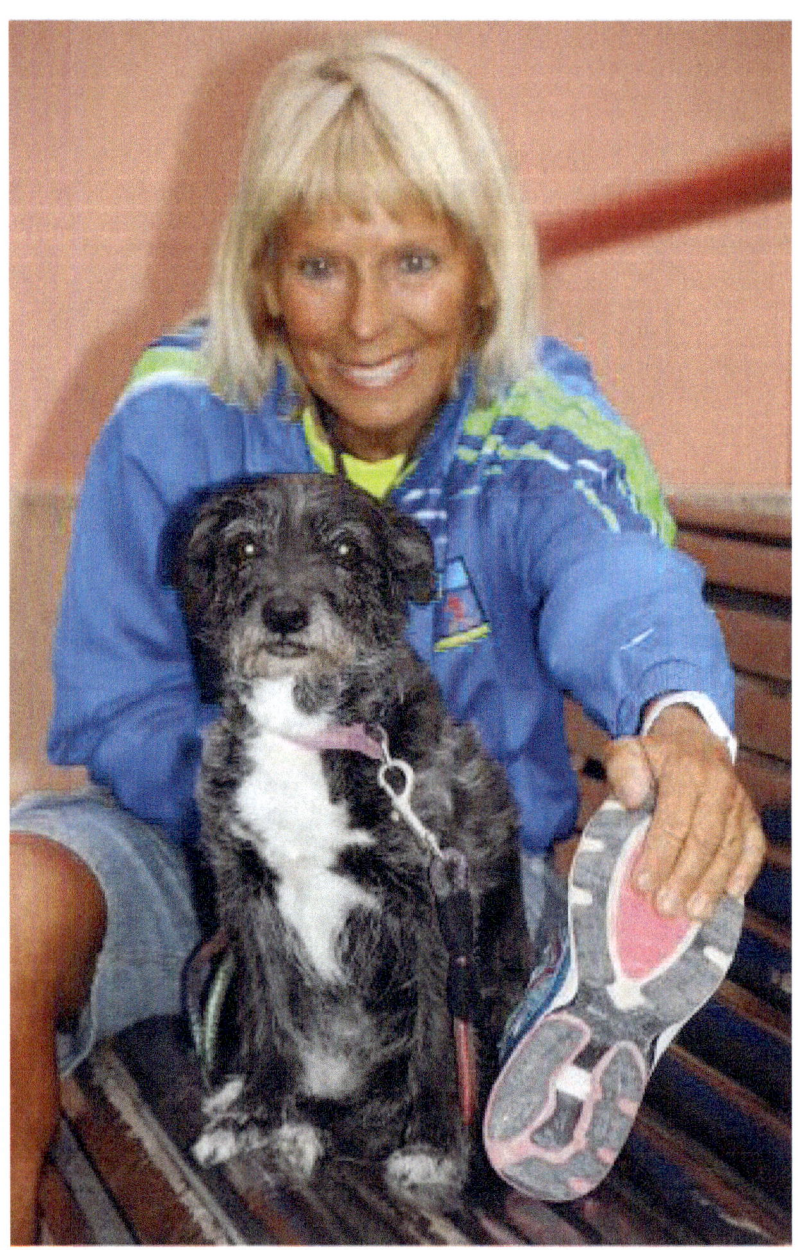

Henriette lived for her running and racing, she was my senior running buddy at 71!

Louise, my running friend, thought she'd impress our beach yoga class by attempting a split for the first time since high school. "Let's just say the only thing I successfully split was my confidence and leggings," she jokes.

Last Thoughts and Recovery

Remember, warming up is about preparing your body for action while lightening the mood. It's a chance to remind yourself that fitness is as much about enjoyment as it is about effort. So swing those arms, shake out those legs, and don't be afraid to laugh at yourself along the way. After all, fitness over 60 is about working smarter, not harder, and having a darn good time while you're at it. It's tempting to power through workouts when you're feeling good, but rest is where the magic happens. Recovery isn't just for elite athletes, it's for anyone who wants to avoid overtraining and stay consistent. Even for the fitter ladies reading this everything has a cycle so if you followed my guide so far things may take longer to build up to tiredness which can be as much as 12 to 13 weeks in my personal experience.

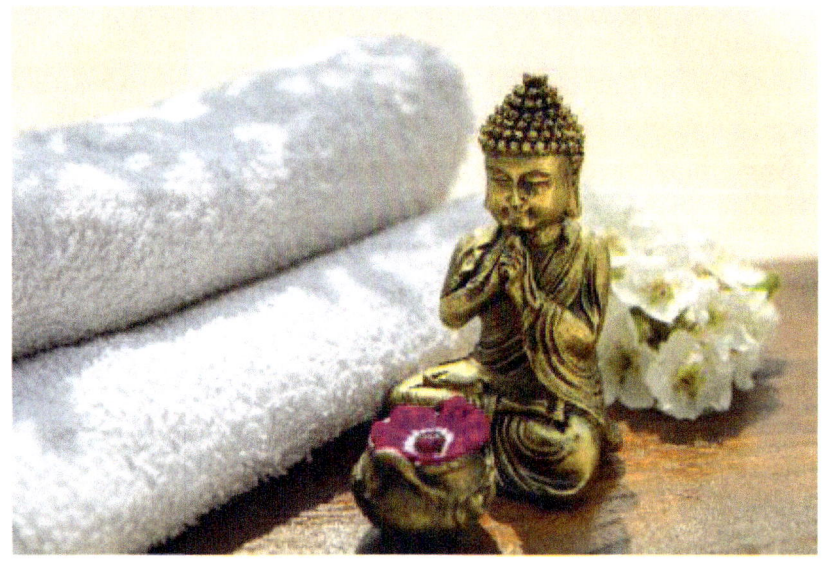

Treat Yourself To a Spa Day and A Relaxing Massage

The signs I have found are a lack of attention, constant tiredness and not wanting to do anything. If that happens take a break and regular walks. Life can build up mentally too I have discovered. Mental energy outage appears to be far more draining on the body than I first ever imagined or simply you've done too much or perhaps races or time in the gym. Book a spa with a relaxing massage for a treat.

Remember your body is there to protect you. I have learned over the years it knows far more than my conscious mind to make decisions for me to listen to. Always listen for that inner voice calling out to me. This applies with the new training regime, if you get any food cravings that are new to you, often it's a depletion of salts, minerals or vitamins that we store within our bodies. Check the craving and research. Discover what is in that product you will be very surprised your body knows what it's lacking so feed it, just not sugars!

Six relaxing ways to help recovery and rest days below that I always plan in my schedule weekly. My favorite is yoga to help relax my mind whilst stretching. I love to incorporate as much into one activity as possible that benefits all of me together to fit into my busy weeks. Dog walking, usually jogging as Kendall is very fast, fast, three times per week.

- Stretching or gentle yoga.
- Swimming
- Walking in the woods (a fan favorite!).
- Listening to your favorite music, while foam rolling (though foam rollers and clumsiness can make for slapstick moments).
- Active house chores or gardening anything that involves paced stretching. You won't even notice, the secret here is to keep going, do not sit around. Muscles ache from good usage and lactic acid buildup.

Drinking plenty of water helps to flush away toxins and repair muscle growth from exercise. I have always found pure beetroot juice to be a great fast healer of tired muscles and I go faster juice 90 minutes before my fitness workouts to energize.

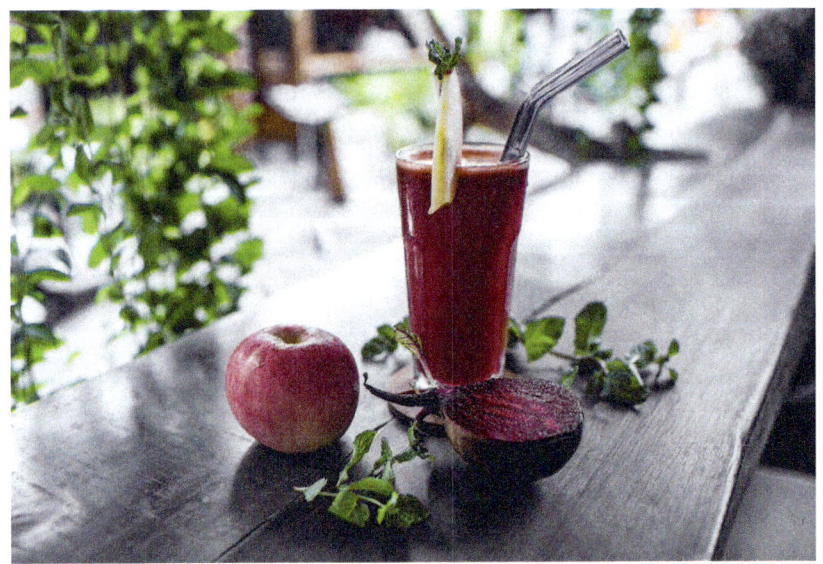

This gorgeous Beetroot smoothie is perfect for fitness activities before and after

Pain vs. Progress. Your body lets you know when you're pushing too hard, it's up to you to listen to those signals.

Good Pain. Soreness from a new workout or challenging your limits.

Bad Pain. Sharp, sudden, or persistent discomfort that means "Stop immediately!"

Tamsin shared how she once mistook muscle soreness for something far worse. "I googled my symptoms and convinced myself I had something wrong with me. Turns out, I'd just used my arms for push-ups for the first time in 30 years."

Staying Flexible – Physically and Mentally. Flexibility isn't just about touching your toes (although that's a great goal). It's also about

adapting your fitness plan when life throws curveballs.
When you're tired, opt for lighter activity instead of skipping exercise altogether. If the weather isn't cooperating, try indoor alternatives like a dance routine or an online yoga class.

Joan said her favorite rainy-day exercise was dancing with her grandchildren to their favorite pop songs. "The moves they taught me were more exhausting than any aerobics class—and ten times more fun!"

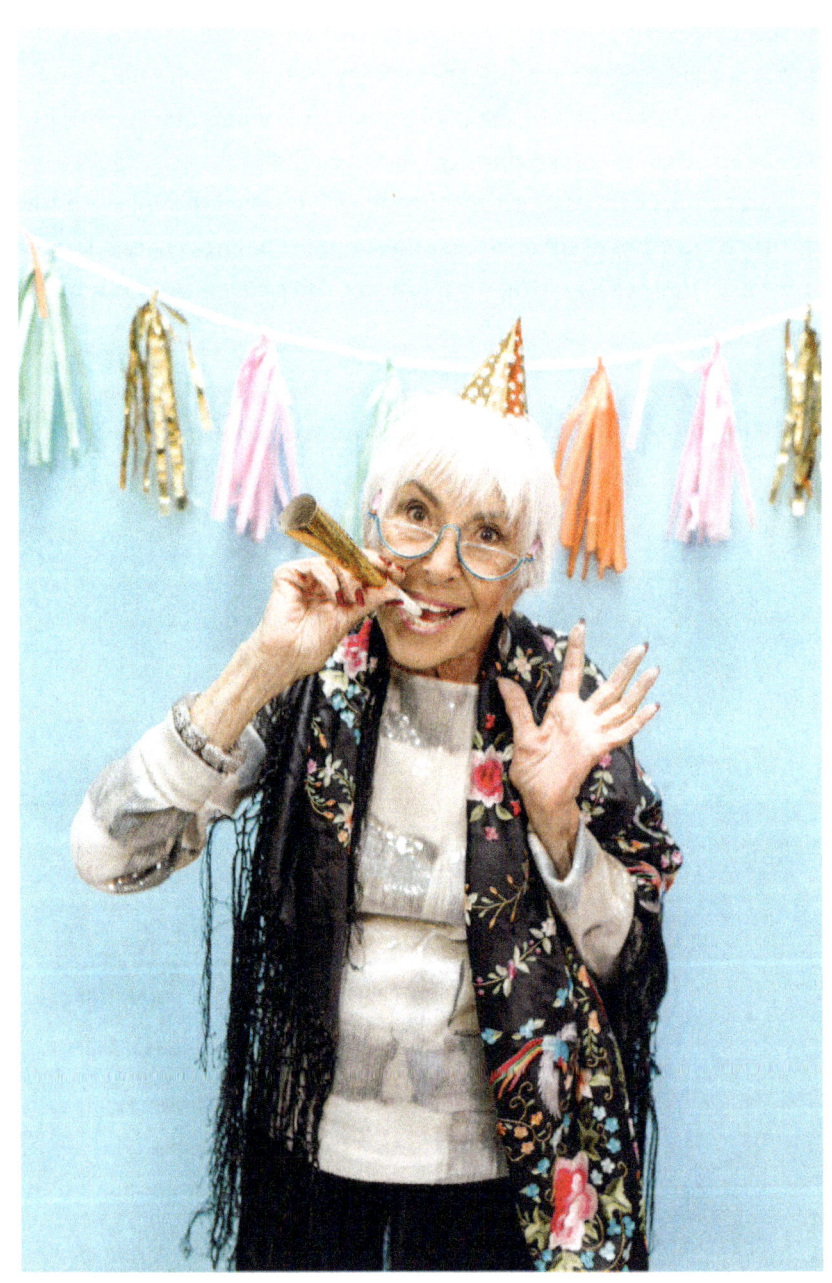

Celebrate Everyday See How Far You Have Come

The Joy of Small Wins. Listening to your body also means celebrating its accomplishments. Every milestone—whether it's walking an extra block or lifting slightly heavier weights—deserves recognition.

- Treat yourself to a massage or spa day.
- Buy new fitness gear (a bright tracksuit or trainers with extra pizzazz).
- Host a "milestone party" with your fitness group.

Weekly Checklist. 5-Step Challenge Stretching Goals

To keep your body flexible and strong this week:

- Start Your Day with Stretching: Dedicate 5 minutes to gentle morning stretches.
- Try Something New: Experiment with a yoga pose you've never done before.
- Stretch During TV Time: Sneak in a hamstring or quad stretch during commercials.
- Stay Consistent: Commit to stretching at least 3 times this week.
- Have Fun: Turn on music, stretch with a friend, or laugh at your "stretch fails."

Conclusion: The Art of Staying Injury-Free

Stretching is more than a physical activity; it's a way to stay connected to your body, reduce stress, and embrace the joys of movement. Over 60, it's not about being perfect; it's about being present.

Stretching teaches patience, perseverance, and humor. Remember, each stretch is a step toward a more physically fit body to regain balance, avoid injury, and build a more confident you. Flexibility is one of the major keys to staying youthful.

Bone-anza! Keeping Those Bones Strong

This chapter dives into why bone health is crucial, especially as we age. Osteoporosis, the silent thief of bone density, becomes a more pressing concern, but the good news is that you can fight back with strength training, proper nutrition, and a little humor.

Did you know your bones are your body's scaffolding? They're the unsung heroes of your anatomy, holding everything up while never demanding a raise. But like any good scaffolding, they need maintenance or you risk them becoming about as sturdy as a house of cards during a sneeze.

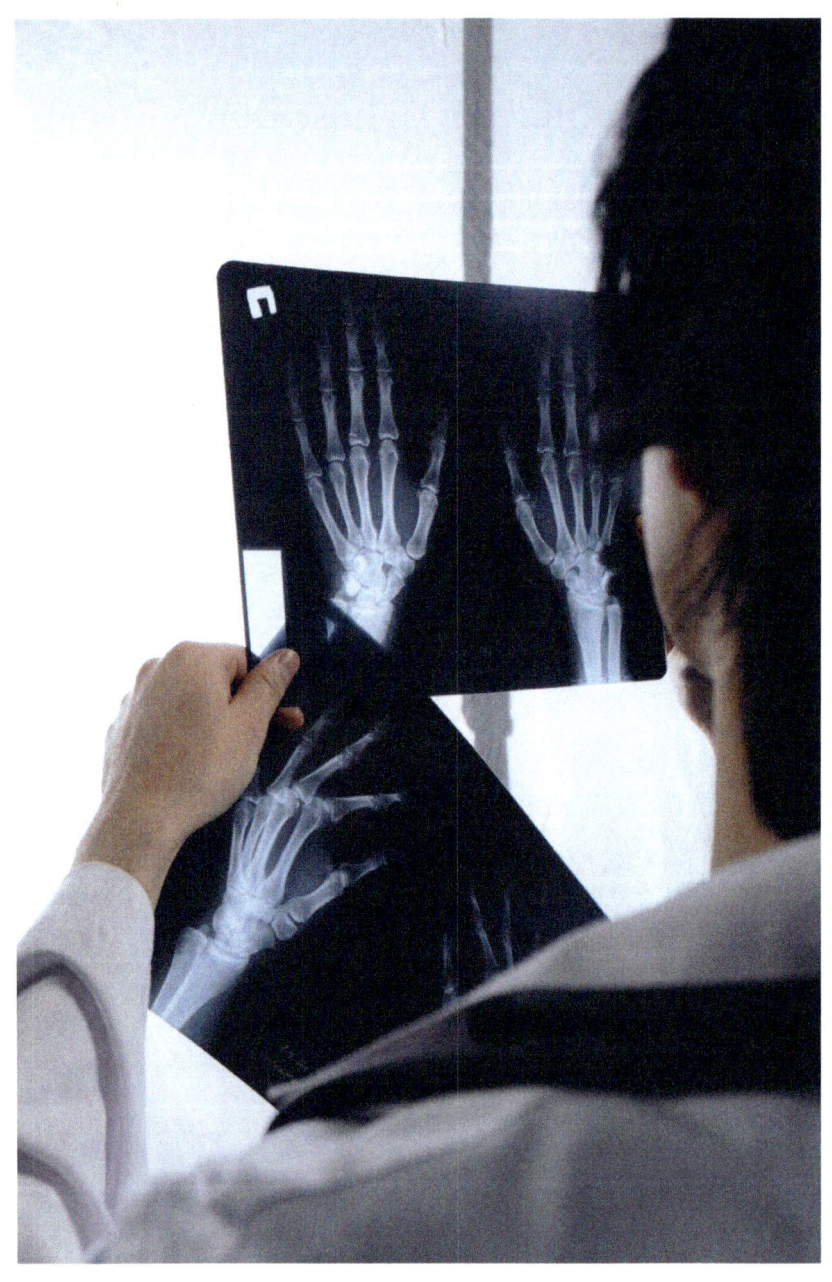

Strong bones provide strength, balance, and support for your body

How to fight osteoporosis with strength training and proper nutrition

Weight-bearing exercises are the secret weapon. Always consult your gym coach for a suitable training program before trying to lift any weights. My shopping bags work well for me walking home as my training.

Imagine this. You're holding a pair of dumbbells. You lift them, feeling like Wonder Woman, minus the lasso and invisible jet. And just as you're about to put them down, you catch your reflection. That's not a tired 60 year old, it's a powerhouse with biceps that could intimidate Popeye. Who needs a knight in shining armor when you've got you?

My son spends more time looking at himself in the gym mirror and making social media videos than he does lifting his weights.

Strengthening your frame for the long haul. "Yoga is about balance—mostly the balance between not falling over and pretending you meant to do that pose."

"It's not about being good at something. It's about being good to yourself"
~ **Unknown**

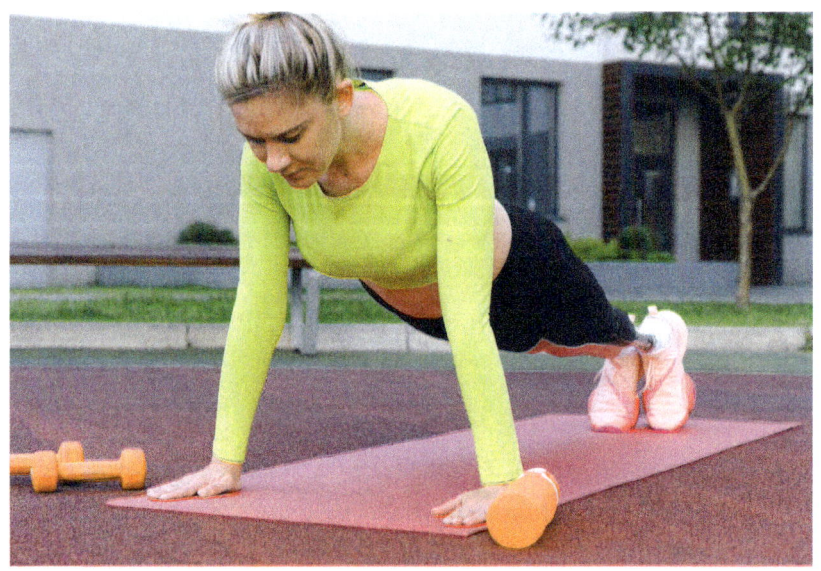

The Plank strengthens the core, increases flexibility, and helps to improve your posture

Your Bones Deserve a Standing Ovation. Bones are the unsung heroes of the body. They're always working hard behind the scenes, supporting you through every movement. By the time you're 60, your bones have been through a lot carrying you through decades of adventures, stumbles, and triumphs. But like any reliable system, they need regular maintenance to keep them strong.

Bone Health 101 – Why It Matters. Bone health isn't just about avoiding fractures it's about maintaining independence and mobility. This is super important to me as an athlete. I have seen many fellow runners with foot stress fractures, which are very painful indeed. After all, who doesn't want to dance at their grandchild's wedding or climb a ladder to sneak a cookie off the top shelf?

Key Facts About Bones: Bone density naturally decreases with age, especially in postmenopausal women. Weight-bearing exercises and strength training are your best defense. Calcium and vitamin D are essential building blocks for bone health. Your skeleton renews itself every 7–10 years, so it's never too late to start improving!

Fun Task. Write down everything you eat daily for each meal or snack in your journal, this is essential to how you feel, train, and watch the calorie intake in my experience of years preparing for races and endurance trails. Reward yourself with a calcium-rich treat like a cheesy omelet or a scoop of natural Greek yogurt.

Lifting Your Spirits (and Weights). Strength training is one of the most effective ways to improve bone density, and you don't need to become a bodybuilder to reap the benefits. A pair of dumbbells, a resistance band, or even a sturdy can of soup can do wonders at home, even carrying the shopping bags home.

Top Tips for Strength Training:

1. Start small: Light weights or bodyweight exercises are a perfect beginning.
2. Focus on consistency over intensity, slow and steady wins the bone race.
3. Target key areas: hips, spine, and wrists are common fracture zones.
4. Mix it up with fun activities like Yoga/Pilates classes or resistance-band workouts.
5. Always warm up and cool down to prevent injuries with stretching too.

Nutrition for Strong Bones:

Building strong bones isn't just about exercise, it's also about what you put on your plate. Sure, you could chug milk like you're auditioning for the '90s "Got Milk?" ad, but let's be real: We're here for solutions that don't make us lactose's latest victim. Instead, think leafy greens, fortified cereals, or (my favorite) a sunny stroll with a side of coffee—calcium in the mug, vitamin D in the sunlight. See? Multitasking!

Bone-Boosting Superfoods:

1. Dairy: Milk, cheese, and yogurt are classic calcium powerhouses.
2. Leafy greens: Kale, spinach, and broccoli pack a calcium punch.
3. Fatty fish: Salmon and sardines are rich in vitamin D.
4. Nuts and seeds: Almonds and sesame seeds are bone-friendly snacks.
5. Fortified foods: Many cereals and juices are fortified with calcium and vitamin D.

Fun Task. Create a "bone-anza" meal plan for one day, featuring at least three bone-friendly foods. Share it with a friend or family member for extra accountability.

Everyday Bone-Saving Habits

Small changes in your daily routine can have a big impact on your bone health with **5 Simple Habits for Stronger Bones:**

1. Take the stairs whenever possible. It's a great weight-bearing exercise.
2. Spend 15 minutes in the sun daily for a natural dose of vitamin D.
3. Practice balance exercises like standing on one foot while brushing your teeth.

4. Quit smoking and limit alcohol intake; both can weaken bones over time.
5. Get a bone density test to stay informed about your progress.

Weekly Checklist: Bone-anza Challenge

Here's your 5-step challenge for building stronger bones this week:

1. Try a New Strength Exercise: Pick a simple movement, like wall push-ups or squats.
2. Add a Bone-Friendly Food: Include one extra calcium-rich food in your daily diet.
3. Soak Up the Sun: Spend 15 minutes outside every day this week.
4. Practice Balance: Try standing on one leg while folding laundry or doing dishes.
5. Celebrate Progress: Write down one thing you did for your bones and share it with a friend or family member.

Conclusion: A Toast to Stronger Bones

Your bones are with you for life, so it's worth investing in them. With a mix of strength training, bone-friendly foods, and a dash of humor, you can keep your skeleton strong and resilient.

Because it's important to laugh too. After her first bone density test, Margaret proudly told her family, "The doctor says my bones are as strong as steel." Her grandson quickly replied, "Does that mean you are part robot now?" Kids love them, they never fail to make me laugh.

Remember, every small step you take whether it's lifting a dumbbell, eating a handful of almonds, or simply soaking up the sun brings you closer to a stronger, healthier you. So go ahead and give your bones the care (and applause) they deserve!

Cardio, Finding Your Groove-Keep Your Heart Happy

The Heart of the Matter

Cardio. The word alone can strike fear into even the most seasoned fitness enthusiast. It conjures up images of endless treadmill runs or aerobics classes that leave you gasping for air like a fish out of water. But cardio doesn't have to be boring, grueling, or torturous. At 60+, it's about finding activities that keep your heart happy while putting a smile on your face.

Your cardiovascular health is essential to longevity and vitality. The good news? You don't have to run marathons to reap the benefits. This chapter explores fun, creative ways to incorporate cardio into your life minus the misery and why keeping your ticker ticking is worth the effort.

Why Cardio Matters:

Cardio, short for cardiovascular exercise, keeps your heart strong, improves circulation, and boosts stamina. It's not just about burning calories, it's about enhancing your overall health.

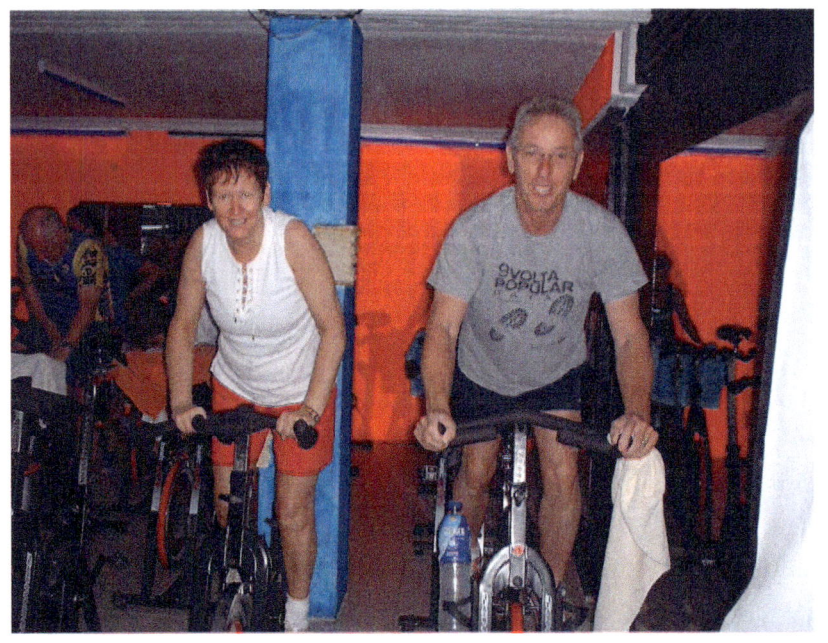

Spinning class in the gym

The Heart of the Matter

Cardio. The word alone can strike fear into even the most seasoned fitness enthusiast. It conjures up images of endless treadmill runs or aerobics classes that leave you gasping for air like a fish out of water. But cardio doesn't have to be boring, grueling, or torturous. At 60+, it's about finding activities that keep your heart happy while putting a smile on your face.

Your cardiovascular health is essential to longevity and vitality. The good news? You don't have to run marathons to reap the benefits. This chapter explores fun, creative ways to incorporate cardio into your life minus the misery and why keeping your ticker ticking is worth the effort.

Why Cardio Matters:
Cardio, short for cardiovascular exercise, keeps your heart strong, improves circulation, and boosts stamina. It's not just about burning calories, it's about enhancing your overall health.

5 Key Benefits of Cardio for Women Over 60:
1. **Heart Health:** Reduces the risk of heart disease and stroke.
2. **Boosts Mood:** Releases endorphins to combat stress and depression.
3. **Enhances Energy:** Improves stamina, making daily tasks easier.
4. **Supports Weight Management:** Helps maintain a healthy weight.
5. **Brain Power:** Improves memory and reduces the risk of cognitive decline.

Fun Task:
Take your pulse before and after a brisk 10-minute walk. Notice the difference and feel proud—you've just given your heart a mini workout!

Cardio doesn't have to mean running circles around the track. Find activities that make your heart happy and keep you coming back for more.

Low-Impact Exercises That Get Your Heart Pumping

Unconventional and I Prefer Fun Cardio Ideas:
1. **Dancing:** From modern jive to salsa, dancing is a fun way to get moving (and maybe meet a partner on the dance floor).
2. **Cycling:** Hop on a bike and explore your local trails. Feel free.
3. **Water Aerobics:** Low impact and high fun, this is perfect for joints.
4. **Walking Guided Tours/Groups:** Discover local landmarks or nature reserves.

5. Hula Hooping: Yes, it's cardio—and it's hilarious!

From Power Walking to Dancing—Who Says Cardio Has to Be Boring?

Walking: The Unsung Hero

Walking is the OG cardio. It's simple, free, and doesn't require Lycra (unless you're into that). Whether it's a brisk stroll around the block or a leisurely walk through the nice warm or air-conditioned mall on hot, rainy, or cold days, every step counts. Bonus: You can window shop and burn calories simultaneously.

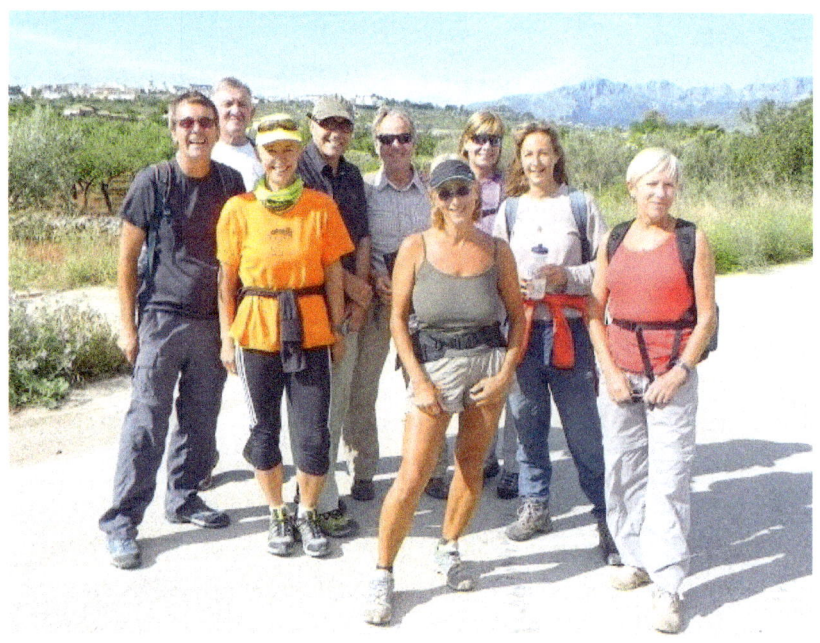

My perfect fitness training day with a trail hike with friends

Dance Your Way to Fitness:
"**When in doubt, dance it out—because sweat looks better with a shimmy.**"

Let's talk cardio: the workout everyone loves to hate. The good news? Cardio doesn't have to mean hours on a treadmill staring at a wall. It's about finding what makes your heart race in the best way—besides a surprise sale at your favorite store.

Dancing Like Nobody's Watching

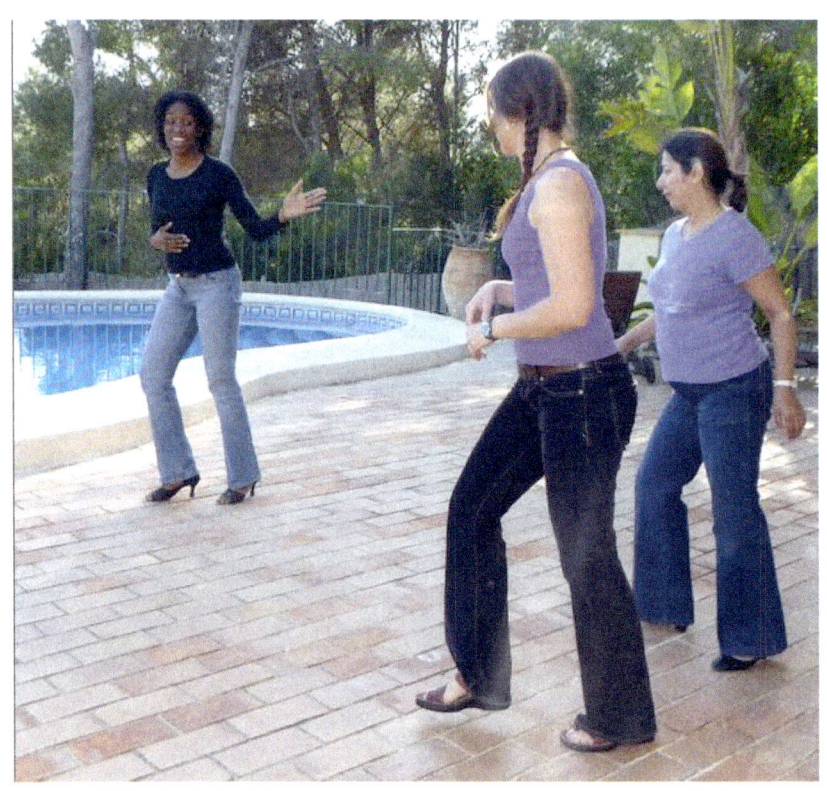

Dancing on holiday is a retreat favorite

Remember the last wedding you went to? The DJ played Dancing Queen, and suddenly your feet were moving like it was 1975. That's cardio, my friend. Zumba, salsa, or even an impromptu living room dance party can count as exercise. Plus, who needs a gym membership when you've got YouTube and a sturdy pair of trainers?

Dance is the hidden language of the soul ~ **Martha Graham**, a dancer and teacher who loved dance

Modern Jive: A Dance for Everyone
　　Modern Jive, also known as Ceroc or Leroc is a fusion of various dance styles, including swing, salsa, and rock and roll. Its straightforward footwork and adaptable nature make it an excellent choice for beginners and seasoned dancers alike. Regular participation can enhance cardiovascular health, improve coordination, and boost mental well-being.

Embarking on a Dance Holiday
　　For a more immersive experience, consider joining a dance holiday abroad. These events offer the opportunity to learn from experienced instructors, enjoy social dancing, and explore new destinations all over the world and all forms of dance. These may include Ballroom, Jive, Latin, Salsa, West Coast Swing, and Country and Western to name a few types of holidays both for couples and singles alike.

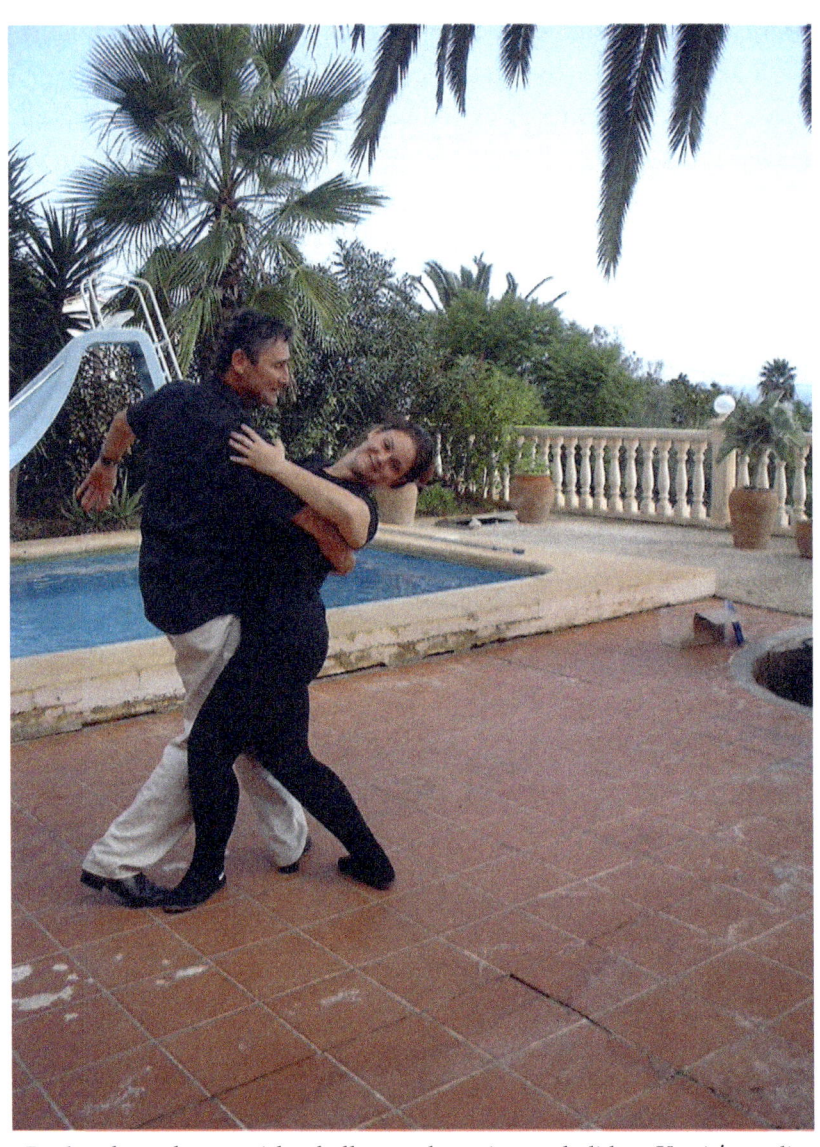

Book a dance lesson with a ballroom champion on holiday. Yes, it's cardio disguised

Benefits of Dance Holidays:

Physical Health & Fitness: Participating in a dance holiday abroad offers numerous benefits: Engaging in daily dance sessions helps maintain and improve physical health.

Mental Well-being: Learning new dance routines and socializing with fellow dancers can enhance cognitive function and reduce stress.

Cultural Exploration: Traveling to new destinations allows you to experience different cultures and environments, enriching your overall experience.

Sam, my sister, thought she'd spice up her cardio routine by trying Zumba. Halfway through, she was convinced the instructor had choreographed the moves just to make her feel like an uncoordinated octopus. "If this is a party," she quipped, "then I'm the guest who showed up three beats too late!"

Cardio, short for cardiovascular exercise, keeps your heart strong, improves circulation, and boosts stamina. It's not just about burning calories—it's about enhancing your overall health.

Beatrice tried hula hooping for the first time since childhood and ended up chasing the hoop around her living room. "Turns out, I'm better at spinning excuses than spinning the hoop," she joked.

Inspirational Story:

At 66, Valerie started jogging 20 minutes daily around her neighborhood. "It's my quiet time," she says. A year later, her doctor was amazed by her blood pressure as it was very low, the doctor asked what she had been doing. When she told him about her training program he remarked he had never seen such a fit senior along with a healthy diet her cholesterol levels passed with flying colors. "Turns out all I needed was trainers and a good playlist," she beams.

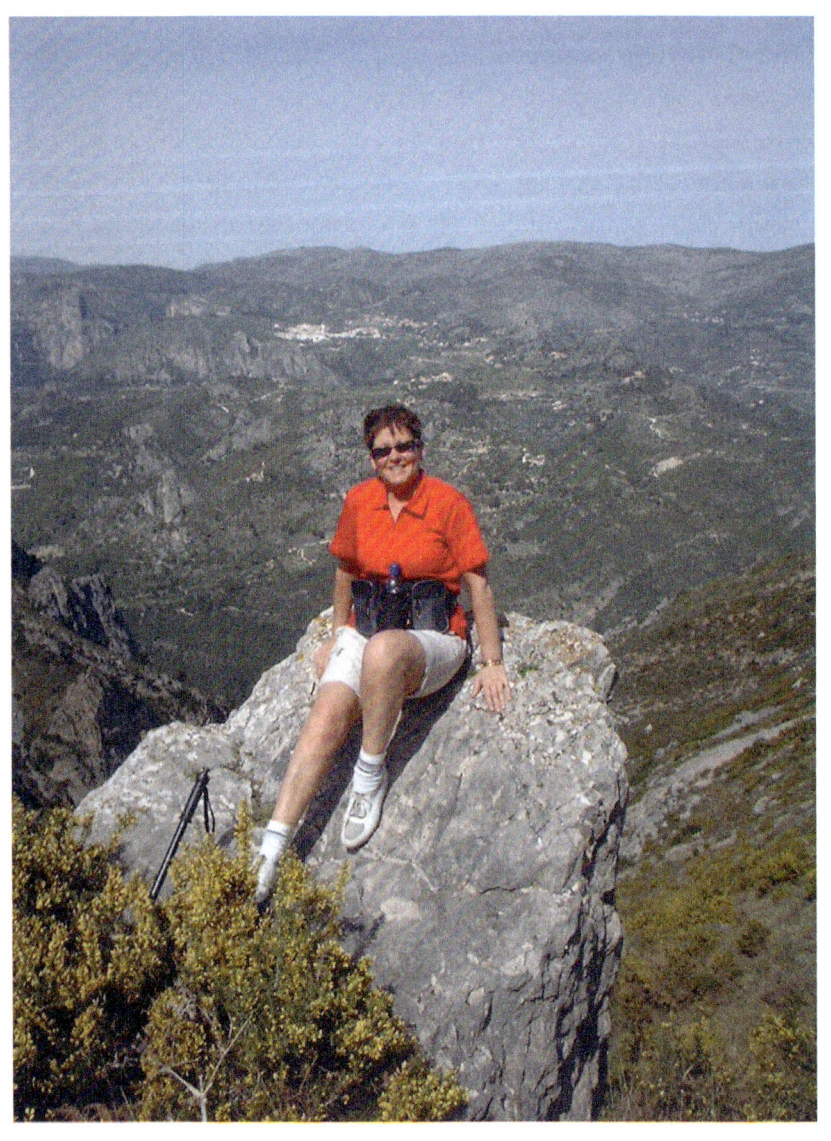

Trail walking can be anywhere you decide

Overcoming the Thought of Cardio:

For many of you, the hardest part of cardio is getting started. The good news is, you don't have to love cardio to benefit from it—find a way to make it enjoyable.

Fun Tips and Tasks to Make Cardio Fun Everywhere

1. Set Small Goals: Start with 5–10 minutes and build up gradually.
2. Find a Buddy: Everything's better with a friend—even sweating.
3. Gamify It: Use apps or trackers to make cardio feel like a game.
4. Mix It Up: Rotate activities to keep things fresh and fun.
5. Reward Yourself: Treat yourself after hitting a cardio milestone—preferably not with cake, no judgment I love Cake too.

Fun Task:
Write a "cardio bucket list" of activities you've always wanted to try, like kayaking or ballroom dancing. Pick one to tackle this month.

Inspirational Story:
Mary, one of my guests from California on her European travels at 70, joined a local walking group with me in Spain to make cardio less boring. "I showed up for the hike with Amanda, but stayed for the gossip after with a cool beer," she laughs. "Now I can't wait to lace up my trainers!" I love Amanda's programs, I never thought fitness could be so much fun with others."

What type of activities should I Choose for Cardio?

Cardio for Every Lifestyle:
Cardio doesn't have to mean setting aside hours for exercise. Sneak it into your daily routine with these easy hacks.

5 Ways to Sneak Cardio Into Your Day:
1. Take the stairs instead of the elevator, it's a mini heart workout.
2. Park farther from the store entrance to get in extra steps.
3. Turn chores into cardio: vacuuming and mopping count!
4. Dance while cooking or doing laundry.
5. Play tag with your grandkids, they'll love it, and so will your heart.

Helen turned her vacuuming into a cardio session by adding lunges. "I got so into it, I forgot to turn the vacuum on," she admits, laughing.

Patricia, 67, realized she could turn her love for gardening into cardio. "Digging, raking, and hauling soil. Who knew getting sweaty in the garden could be so satisfying?"

The secret here is to plan your workout the night before and visualize yourself doing it. Even as a guide, it's second nature to me even dog walking combining my daily hour run. I am not sure who fitter me or the dog Kendall.

Believe it or not but since sitting down to write this fitness book, I get up from my chair to stretch, jog around the kitchen, run upstairs, and refresh my body for the next hour whilst I write with plenty of water. If you are still working a job; as many early seniors still are in these economic times, sitting down thinking how you can work whilst on the work timetable and getting paid for it too!

5-Step Weekly Cardio Weekly Challenge

Here's your 5-step cardio challenge for the week:

1. Try a New Activity: Choose something fun like dancing, cycling, or swimming.
2. Set a Goal: Aim for 30 minutes of cardio 3 times this week (or break it into 10-minute chunks).
3. Track Your Steps: Use a pedometer or app to see how much you move daily.
4. Invite a Friend: Make it social to stay motivated.
5. Celebrate Progress: Reward yourself for completing the challenge—maybe with a relaxing foot soak

Conclusion: The Joy of a Happy Heart

Cardio doesn't have to feel like a chore. When you find activities you love, you're more likely to stick with them—and your heart will thank you for it.

After completing her first 5K walk, Heather proudly declared, "I didn't come in first, but I also didn't call a taxi halfway through. That's what I call a win!"

Remember, every step you take and every beat of your heart is a reminder of your strength and resilience. Whether you're waltzing around your living room or power-walking through the park, keep moving forward—because cardio, you've got this!

Yoga, Pilates, and Pretzel-Like Positions

"Yoga is about balance, mostly the balance between not falling over and pretending you meant to do that pose."

Yoga and Pilates have an unfair reputation for requiring extreme flexibility. But trust me, nobody starts out looking like a human pretzel. Most of us begin looking more like a bent paperclip.

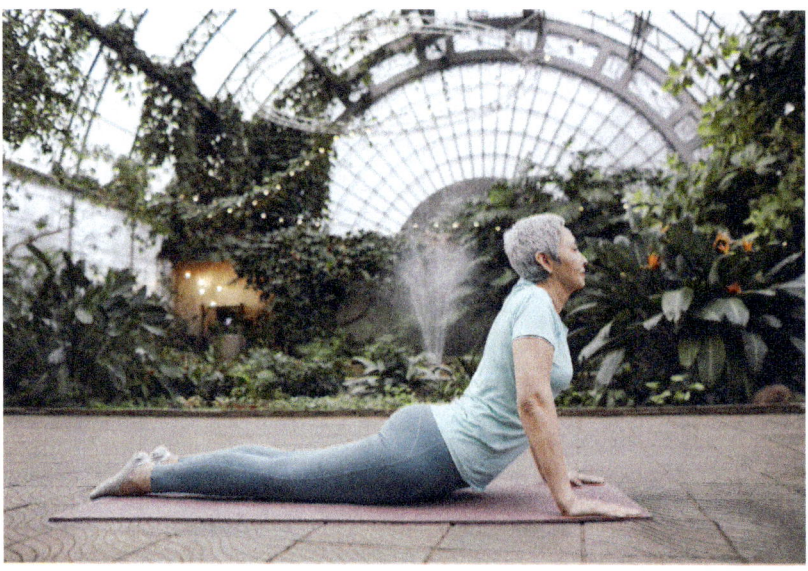

The Cobra Pose

Exploring gentle yoga and Pilates for strength and balance

Yoga: Zen Without the Judgment

Yoga is about balance, breathing, and reminding yourself that it's okay if your "downward dog" looks more like a "napping beagle." Start small with poses like Child's Pose (because, let's be honest, it's mostly lying down) and work your way up.

Pilates: The Core of the Matter

Pilates isn't just about crunches; it's about engaging your core, which is the body's powerhouse. Think of it as the trunk of your tree, a strong core, strong everything else. And if you wobble? That's just you channeling your inner jellyfish.

Finding Balance in More Ways Than One:

Yoga and Pilates are like the dynamic duo of fitness: one focuses on mindfulness and flexibility, while the other builds core strength and stability. Together, they create a powerhouse of benefits for your body and mind. At 60, these practices can improve posture, increase mobility, and even reduce stress. Plus, they give you an excuse to buy stretchy pants and call it self-care.

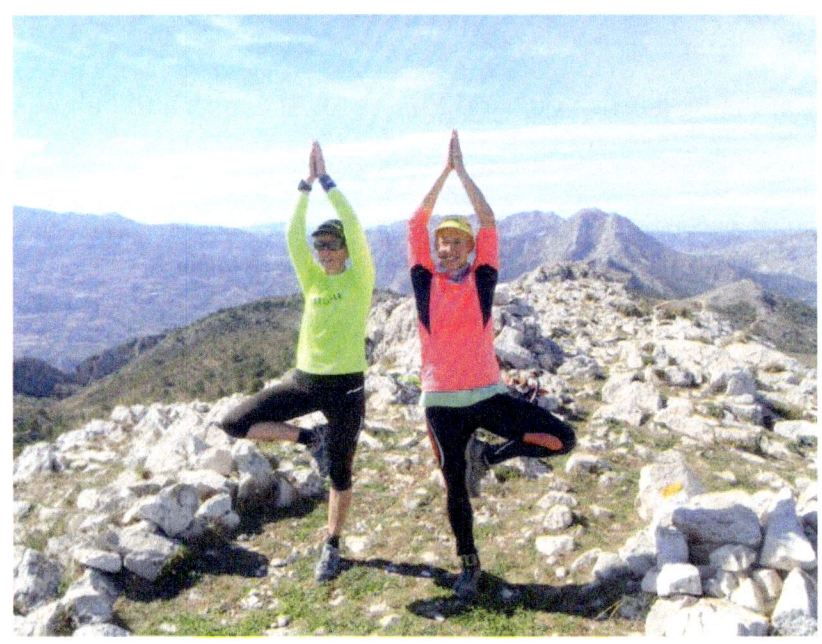

A balance called the Tree Pose fun on the mountain

But let's be honest getting started can feel a bit intimidating. Who hasn't felt a twinge of doubt while eyeing a yoga class full of people twisted into pretzel-like poses? Fear not! This chapter breaks down yoga and Pilates into manageable, enjoyable steps, with a side of humor to keep things light.

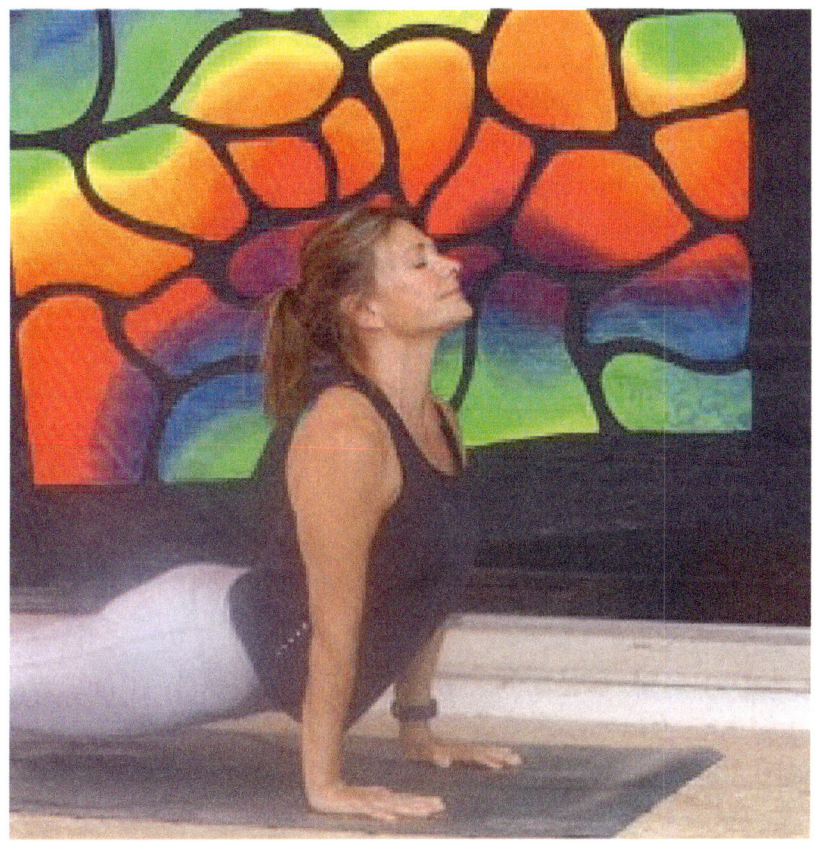

Pure in the zone

At 60+, you've earned the right to embrace yoga, not because it's trendy or because your neighbor swears by it, but because nothing beats the joy of moving your body and finding a little peace amid life's chaos. And let's be real: bending and stretching in ways you didn't know were possible makes you feel like a graceful (if slightly creaky) swan.

Why Yoga is Perfect for Women Over 60

Flexibility with a Side of Grace:
Whether you're reaching for your toes or attempting a downward dog, yoga helps you stretch in ways that remind your body it's still capable of amazing things.

Balance for the Real World:
Tree pose isn't just for Instagram—it's for those moments when the cat darts underfoot, and you need to stay upright.

Stress Relief, One Breath at a Time:
Deep breathing isn't just a yoga thing; it's a life thing. Bonus: it's harder to yell at the TV when you're inhaling for five counts.

The Yoga Mat Chronicles: What to Expect

1. First-Time Yoga Class Nerves
Walking into your first yoga class can feel daunting like entering another world. Everyone's wearing stretchy pants, there's calming music playing, and the instructor keeps saying things like, "Find your inner light."

Translation: Don't overthink it. Everyone's too busy trying not to fall out of warrior pose to notice you wobbling.

2. Learning the Lingo
Downward Dog: Essentially sticking your bum in the air and hoping gravity doesn't betray you.
Savasana: The part where you lie down and pretend to meditate while secretly planning dinner.

3. Your Yoga Superpower:
Flexibility isn't just about touching your toes, it's about adapting.

Modify the poses, use props, and remember: the only competition is with yourself (and maybe the overly bendy 30-something next to you).

3 Quick Yoga Poses for Home

1. Cat-Cow Stretch
Start on all fours. Arch your back (cow), then round it (cat).
Why: It's great for the spine and gets those creaky joints moving.
Bonus: It feels oddly empowering to moo and meow if no one's watching.

2. Chair Pose (with a Chair)
Stand behind a sturdy chair and hold onto the backrest. Bend your knees slightly, as if sitting in an imaginary chair.
Why: Strengthens thighs and improves balance.
Bonus: Imagine you're lowering yourself onto a throne—it's all about mindset.

3. Seated Forward Fold
Sit on the floor with your legs straight out. Reach for your toes, or as close as you can get.
Why: Stretches the hamstrings and releases tension in the lower back.
Bonus: It's the perfect time to reminisce about your flexibility in your twenties.

Zen Moments for Real Life
Yoga isn't just about poses; it's about mindfulness. Try these yoga-inspired practices:

Breathe Before You React: Whether it's a snarky comment or a frustrating day, take a deep breath before responding. You'll feel calmer—and you'll win the argument.

Stretch Anytime, Anywhere: Long car rides? Stretch your neck. Waiting in line? Do a subtle calf raise. (Okay, maybe not so subtle—own it!)

Find Joy in the Present: Whether it's a cup of tea or a sunrise, yoga practice reminds us to savor life's little moments.

The Real Joy of Yoga

Yoga isn't about becoming a human pretzel; it's about moving, breathing, and laughing at yourself along the way. So grab your mat, embrace the wobble, and enjoy the journey—Zen doesn't care if you giggle during meditation.

Remember yoga is for life and that it cannot solve all your issues or stress in one yoga retreat or class. Like everything in life, it is the practice of constant self-improvement. It's about meeting yourself where you are and growing from there. For senior women 60+ and older, yoga offers countless benefits, from improved flexibility to a calmer mind.

Fun Task:

Look up a free beginner yoga class online and try it out this week. Bonus if you make it through without giggling during Savasana. Check out classes online for your holidays.

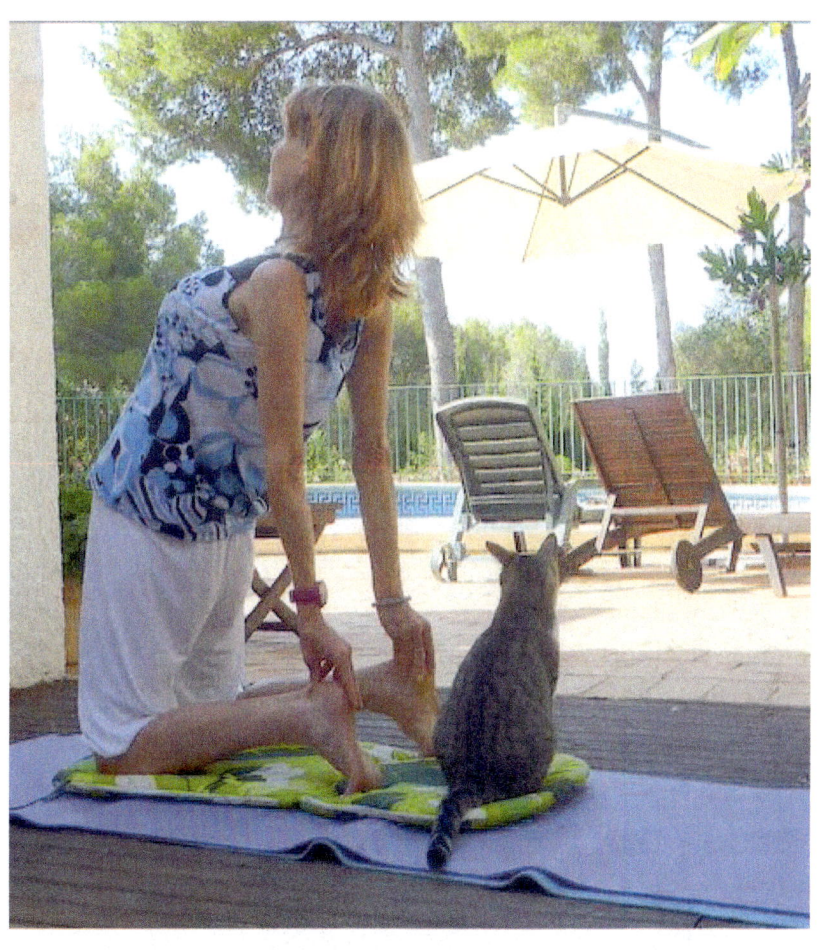

Yoga kitty Isabelle cannot wait to sit on Louise's mat

Weekly Checklist: The Yoga Challenge

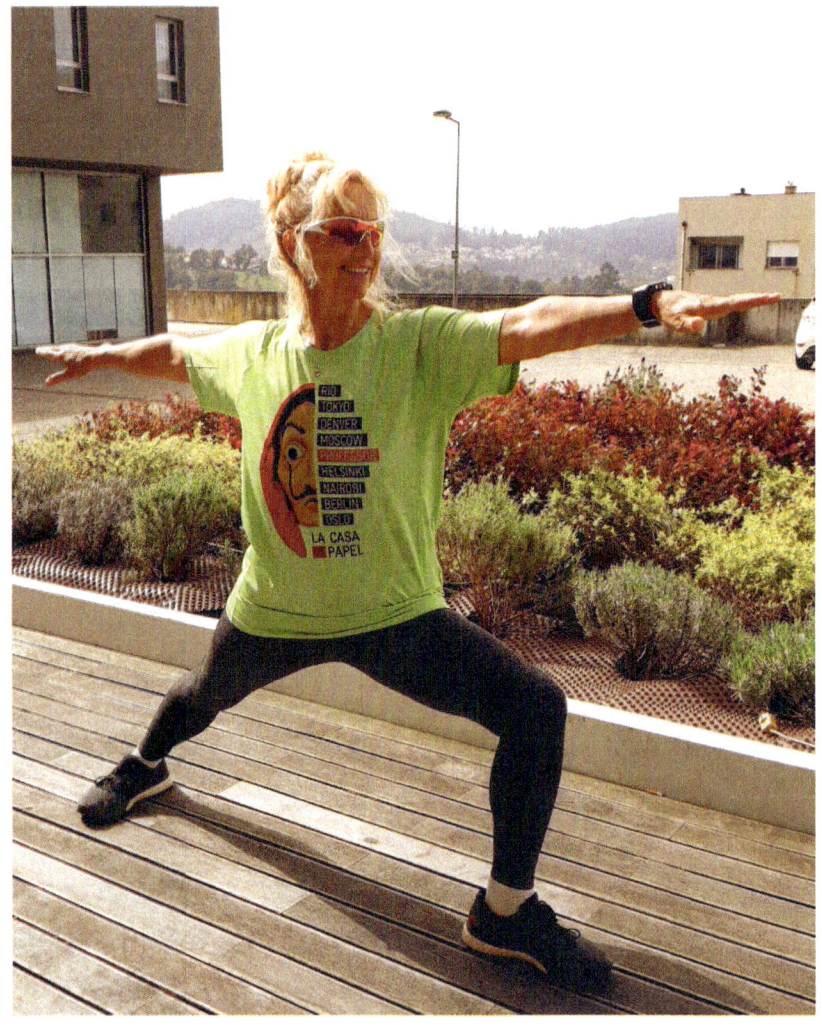

The dynamic Warrior Pose in Portugal on holiday

Ready to bring yoga into your life? Here's your 5-step challenge for the week:

1. **Try One New Pose:** Choose a beginner pose and practice it daily.
2. **Breathe Deeply:** Spend 5 minutes practicing a breathing technique.
3. **Attend a Class:** Join a local or online session to learn from an instructor.
4. **Create a Routine:** Commit to 10 minutes of yoga every day.
5. **Celebrate Your Progress:** Treat yourself to a calming tea or a yoga-inspired playlist.

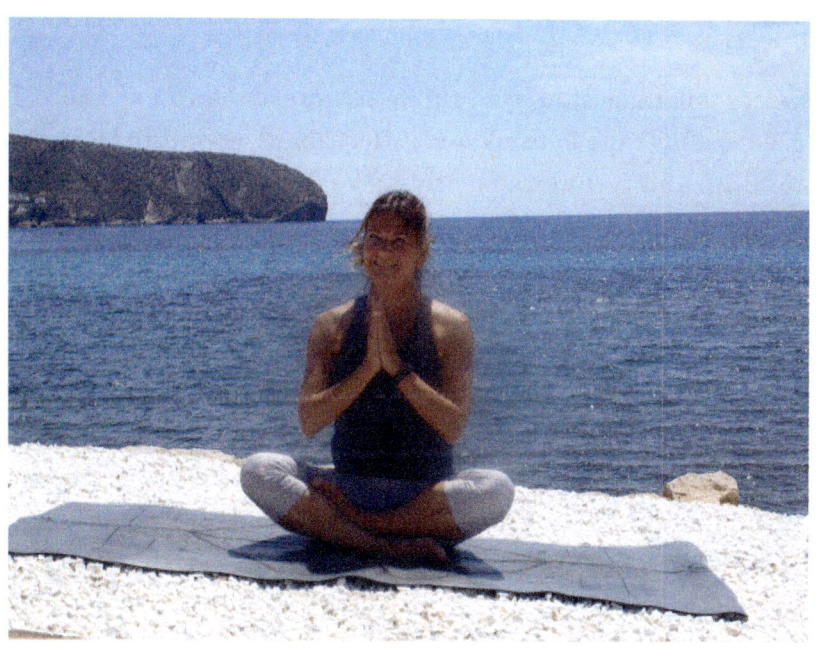

Yoga on the beach with my instructor also called Amanda

Conclusion: Stretching Toward Joy

Yoga isn't about perfection, it's about progress, patience, and finding joy in the journey. Whether you're mastering your Warrior Pose or simply enjoying a few moments of deep breathing, every effort counts.

Remember, yoga is a gift to yourself, a chance to move, breathe, and laugh at life's quirks. Embrace it with an open heart and a sense of humor, and you'll find that inner peace is just a stretch away.

Here's What Claire from Scotland had to say about the benefits of yoga and mindfulness while at my retreat how she felt and the takeaway benefits.

" **Dear Amanda, I enjoyed this week more than I expected. It gave me lots time to think and reflect about my future and learn to think and feel more positive. I really enjoyed the yoga and mindfulness sessions. I loved the food and new ways of cooking. I am going back a more positive person." - Thanks Claire**

Learn the word Namaste. You will hear it spoken many times over in classes wherever you are.

Namaste comes from ancient Sanskrit and means " bowing to you" or " I bow to you" with hands in the prayer position used often as a thank you to your instructor at the end of the class following your Shavasana time on the mat or meeting fellow yogis on your travels.

Strength Training for Senior Superwomen

It's time to talk about lifting weights. Don't panic, this isn't about becoming the next bodybuilder grunting on the cover of Muscle Monthly. Strength training at 60+ is about becoming the superhero version of yourself: strong, steady, and capable of opening jars without calling in reinforcements.

"Lifting weights over 60 doesn't make you old-school, it makes you hardcore."

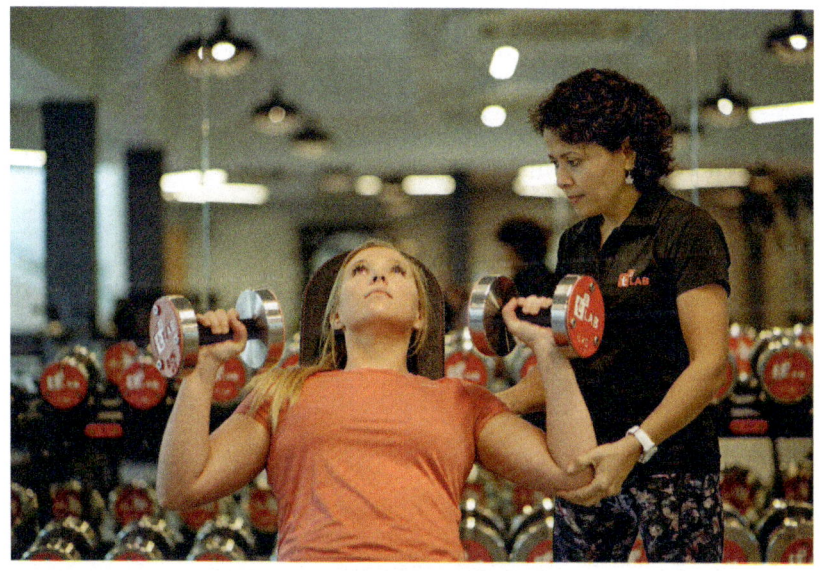

Always ask the trainer at the Gym for a program to suit your level

The Lighter Side of Lifting

"Weights don't judge, but they will remind you that you skipped arm day last week."
   Let's face it, life is heavy. From lugging groceries to wrangling grandkids, there's always something to lift, carry, or move. The good news? Strength training doesn't just prepare you for life's physical demands, it gives you the confidence to tackle them head-on. Plus, let's be honest, nothing beats the satisfaction of flexing your biceps in the mirror and thinking, Well, hello, muscles!

Why Strength Training?

Strength training isn't just about muscles. It's about independence. It's about carrying your groceries, standing tall, and shooing away the occasional spider without a second thought. Plus, it's one of the best ways to help keep osteoporosis at bay and improve your balance because nobody wants to reenact a slapstick comedy fall in real life or be seen on social media in a funny viral video.

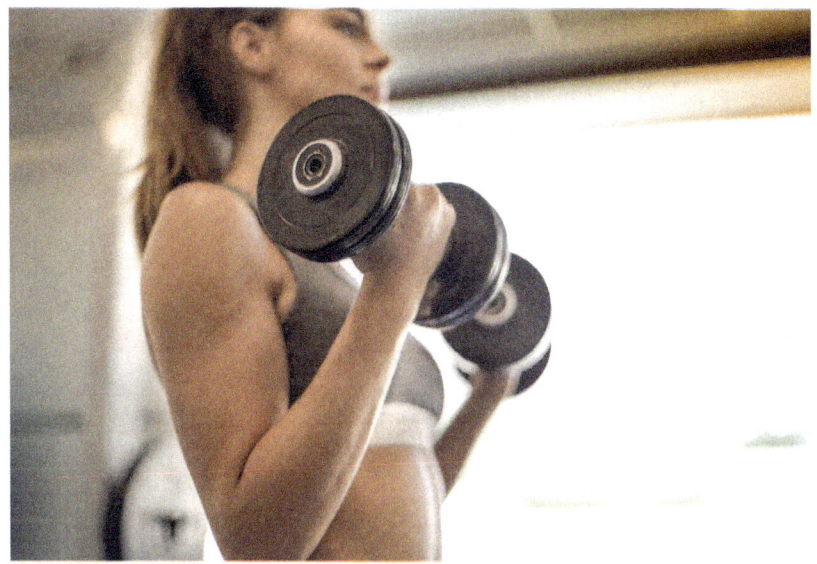

Be kind To yourself it's not a race, just be consistent with a weekly routine

The Benefits of Strength Training:

- Build Bone Density:
- Each time you lift a weight, your bones get the memo: "Oh, she means business. Better fortify!"
- Translation: You're keeping osteoporosis on its toes while staying off yours.
- Boost Balance and Coordination:

Strength training can help you stay upright in moments of chaos, like when your dog spots a squirrel mid-walk and does that cartoon bit with back legs spinning out before launching itself like a rocket full charge with you trying to hang on. Yikes!

Feel Like a Total Badass:

Carrying all the groceries in one trip? Crushing pickle jars without assistance? That's the strong-you glow.

My First Encounter with Dumbbells:

I'll never forget my first day with dumbbells. They were pink and cute, and I thought, How hard could this be? Ten minutes later, I was sweating hard, but I felt like a champion. The thing about strength training is that it sneaks up on you, you start light, maybe with soup cans, and before you know it, you're lifting weights heavier than your handbag. Just get your favorite tunes blasting at full tilt, forget the neighbors for an hour, and just do it.

5 Simple Strength Routines for Home and My Tips

Let's Get Started:

1. Chair Squats: Sit and stand from a chair, pretending you're about to win an award for "Best Squat Form in a Sitcom."

Why: They strengthen your legs and glutes, helping you stand up, sit down, and dance like nobody's watching.

How: Stand in front of a chair, feet shoulder-width apart.

Lower yourself until your bottom just touches the seat.

Stand back up. (Bonus points if you do it without using your hands!)

Reps: 10-15, or until you feel the burn. Go for 3 sets building slowly over time as it begins to get easier with no soreness.

Pro Tip: If you start giggling halfway through because it feels like musical chairs, you're doing it right.

Muscles worked: Legs, glutes.

Tip: Keep a sturdy chair nearby (no wobbly antiques).

2. **Wall Push-Ups:** Lean against a wall and push yourself away. It's like a regular push-up but without the drama of lying on the floor.
Why: Great for arms and chest without requiring you to lie on the floor. (Because let's be honest, getting back up is half the battle.)
How: Stand facing a wall. Place your hands flat on it, shoulder-width apart.
Lean forward, keeping your body straight, then push back.
Reps: 8-12. Aim for 3 sets. Build up over a month.
Pro Tip: Pretend the wall is your annoying neighbor. Push hard.
Muscles worked: Arms, chest.
Tip: Whisper, "I'm stronger than yesterday," for bonus motivation.

3. **Bicep Curls:** Grab light weights (or water bottles) and curl them up toward your shoulders. Feel free to strike a pose, it's part of the workout.
Why: Toned arms are fabulous for sleeveless tops and opening jars like a pro.
How: Hold a water bottle (or a 2-3 lb dumbbell) in each hand.
Keep your elbows close to your sides and curl the weights up to your shoulders. Lower slowly.
Reps: 10-12. Work towards building 3 sets over time.
Pro Tip: Imagine the weights are tiny trophies celebrating how amazing you are.
Muscles worked: Arms.
Tip: Avoid the temptation to use wine bottles as lifting them might give you other ideas.

4. **Standing Calf Raises:** Hold onto a chair for balance and lift your heels off the ground. Repeat until you feel taller (or at least stronger).

Why: Strengthen your calves and improve your balance. Plus, they make you feel taller (or at least closer to your favorite high shelf).

How: Stand tall and hold onto a chair for support.

Slowly lift your heels off the ground, then lower.

Reps: 10-15. Aim for 3 sets eventually.

Pro Tip: If you're feeling extra fancy, grab a feather boa and imagine you're strutting down a runway.

Muscles worked: Calves.

Tip: Imagine you're reaching for something on the top shelf.

5. Plank on the Wall (Or Table):

Coffee table or the dining room table, even a strong chair, or perhaps your local park bench.

Why: A strong core helps with everything—from balance to back health to standing tall.

How: Place your hands flat on a sturdy table or wall, step back, and keep your body straight up.

Hold for 10-20 seconds, gradually increasing over time.

Pro Tip: Distract yourself by singing a song—Eye of the Tiger works wonders.

Muscles Worked: This is for your "six-pack" muscle, crucial for stabilizing your core and maintaining proper posture during the plank. Providing core strength and stability to help prevent falls. Also, the deltoids which are your shoulder muscles that heavily support your upper body, again help to maintain posture and balance.

Tip: If you're with a friend, challenge them to a "plank-off" and see who can hold it longer. The winner gets to pick the next exercise!

My Closing Pep Talk Ladies:

Remember, strength training isn't about looking like someone else. It's about becoming the strongest, happiest, most capable version of you. You don't need to lift heavy weights to feel powerful, you just need to show up, try your best, and keep at it.

The Only Bad Workout is the one you didn't miss!

Strength Training Myths Busted

Myth #1: Strength Training is for Bodybuilders.
Nope! It's for anyone who wants to stay independent and feel like a rockstar in their daily life.

Myth #2: I Need Fancy Equipment.
False. You've got a built-in gym at home, the park, and in nature anywhere really, a tree works too. Chairs, water bottles, and even your body weight can work wonders.

Myth #3: I'm Too Old for This.
Excuse me? Grandma Moses started painting at 78, and you're telling me you're "too old" to pick up a 3 lb dumbbell? Nonsense.

Signs You're Crushing It

Your arms don't jiggle quite as much when you wave.

You can carry all the groceries at once and the neighbours are impressed.

You feel a little taller, stronger, and prouder every single day.

Will I get bulky?:
A very good question indeed and most commonly asked.

Not unless you're lifting tractor tires. For most women, strength training tones and defines muscles, helping you look and feel fabulous. Start light, listen to your body, and focus on form. It's about progress, not perfection. And if you drop a dumbbell? Just say it was part of the plan.

What if I hurt myself?:

Start light, listen to your body, and focus on form. It's about progress, not perfection. And if you drop a dumbbell? Just say it was part of the plan.

The Emotional Payoff:
The best part of strength training isn't just physical. It's the moment you realize you're getting stronger, both inside and out. Maybe it's the day you lift a bag of potting soil without breaking a sweat. Or the moment you look in the mirror and see a hint of definition in your arms.

Conclusion: You are Superwoman in Every Way

Remember, darling, you're not training to look a certain way you're training to feel a certain way: strong, capable, and confident ready to take on the world (or at least the nearest flight of stairs). Suddenly, challenges feel smaller, and possibilities feel endless. You're not just lifting weights; you're lifting yourself into a version of yourself that's unstoppable.

So grab those weights, strike your best superhero pose in your mirror, and say it with me: I am a Superwoman!

The Art of Falling Gracefully (and Avoiding It)

At 60+, falling takes on a new significance. It's not just about avoiding a scraped knee, it's about ensuring you bounce back (preferably without too much creaking). The truth is, falling isn't something to fear; it's something to prepare for. With improved balance, awareness, and a sense of humor, even the occasional tumble can become less intimidating.

This chapter is dedicated to mastering the art of staying upright, minimizing injuries, and yes, even falling with flair when gravity has other plans. We'll share practical tips, exercises, and real-life stories to help you build confidence and resilience, proving that no matter what, you can get back up—physically and mentally.

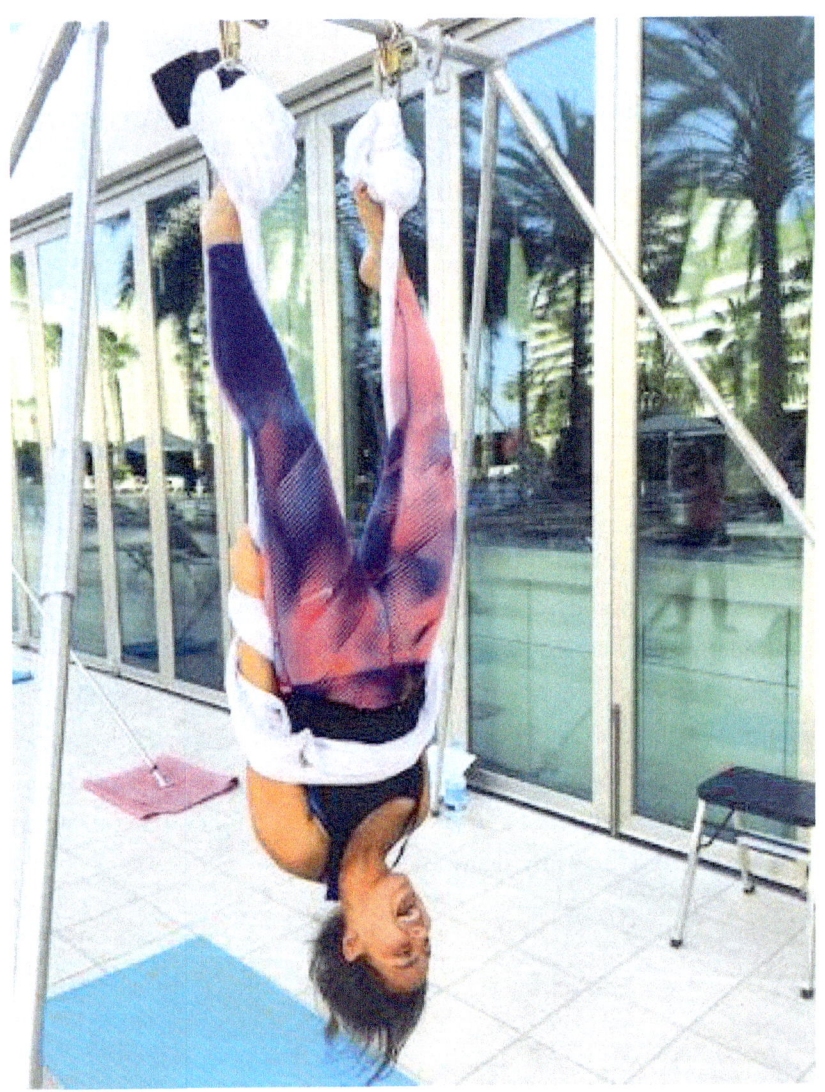

Aerial yoga is popular in Spain

First, let's clear something up: If you've tripped recently, it's not because you're "getting old." It's because gravity is a petty little force that plays no favorites. But fear not—balance exercises can make you more stable than a Zen monk at a rock concert.

The Balance Challenge:
Here's a fun way to test your balance: Stand on one leg while trying to fold laundry. Bonus points if you don't knock over the dog. Why? Because life is full of unexpected wobbles, and a little practice can keep you upright when they come your way.

Why Balance Matters More Than Ever

Balance isn't just for tightrope walkers. As we age, our ability to maintain stability naturally declines, increasing the risk of falls. But the good news is that balance can be improved with consistent effort.

Life is a balance of holding on and letting go
  ~ **Rumi**

The Perks of Better Balance:

1. **Fall Prevention:** Reduces the likelihood of accidents.
2. **Increased Confidence:** You'll feel more secure in your movements.
3. **Improved Posture:** Helps you stand tall and move gracefully.
4. **Enhanced Mobility:** Makes everyday activities easier.
5. **Boosts Brain Health:** Balance exercises engage the mind and body.

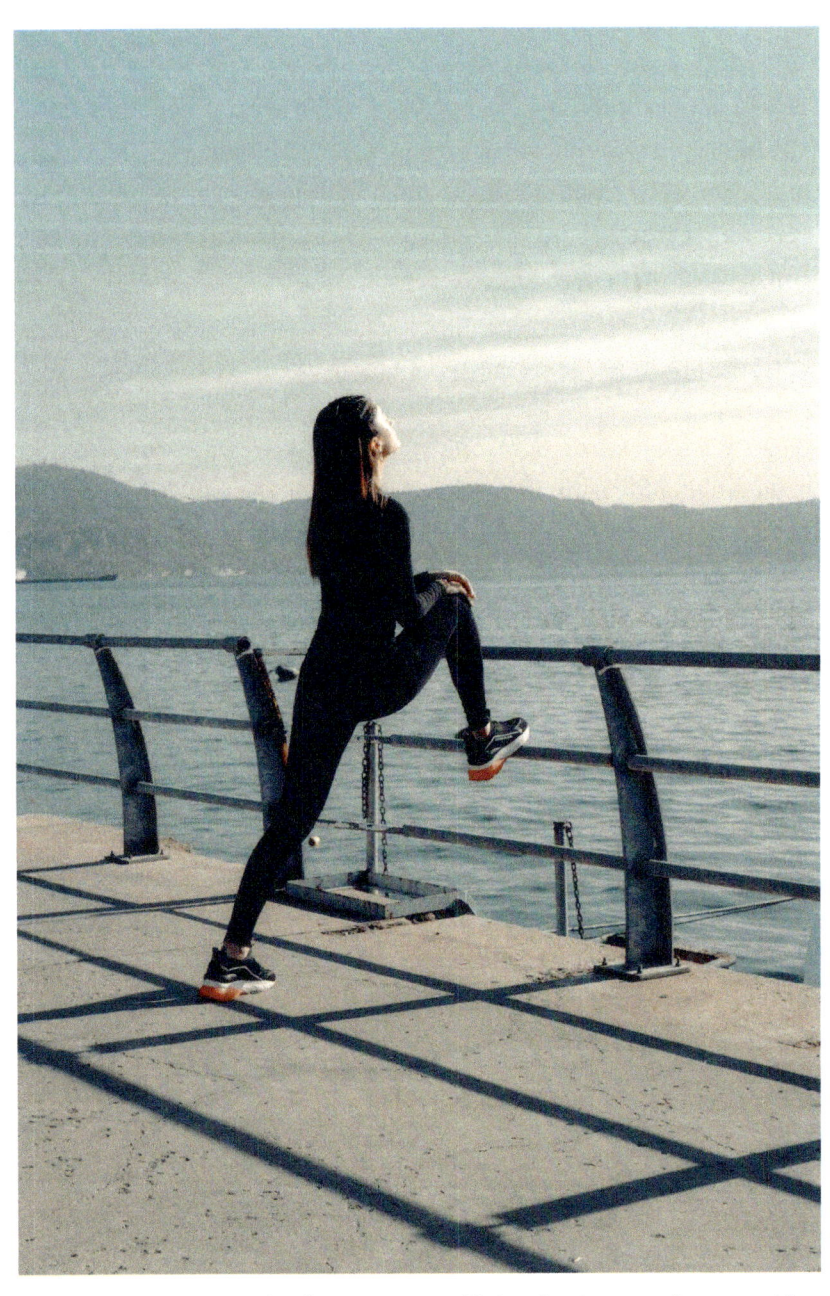

Stretch, balance, and reflect in nature. Enjoy the time out for yourself

Fall Stories: Laugh Through the Bruises

We all have that one fall story that's equally hilarious and mortifying. Mine involved a banana peel, yes, like a cartoon, and an audience of teenagers. But the silver lining? I realized I needed to work on balance, and now I can plank longer than they can text.

Fun Task:

Stand on one leg while brushing your teeth. If you wobble, blame it on the toothpaste.

Exercises to Improve Balance

Improving balance doesn't require fancy equipment or gym memberships. A few simple exercises can make a big difference.

Top Balance Exercises:

1. **Tightrope Walk:** Walk heel-to-toe in a straight line, like you're on a tightrope.
2. **Tree Pose:** A classic yoga pose that builds stability and focus.
3. **Single-Leg Stands:** Hold onto a chair for support and gradually increase the time you balance on one foot.
4. **Rock the Boat:** Stand with your feet hip-width apart, and shift your weight from one side to the other.
5. **Toe Lifts:** Stand on your toes, hold for a few seconds, then lower back down.

Humorous Anecdote:

Helen tried the tree pose in her kitchen and ended up hugging the fridge for support. "I wasn't falling, I was just really attached to my leftovers!"

Fun Task:

Try walking across the room while balancing a book on your head. Extra points if it's a fitness book, you're now living with me.

The Art of Falling Safely

Despite your best efforts, falls happen. The key is knowing how to fall safely to minimize injury.

Tips for Falling Gracefully:

1. **Don't Fight It:** Trying to resist a fall often makes it worse.
2. **Tuck and Roll:** Protect your head by tucking your chin and rolling to distribute impact.
3. **Land on the Fleshy Bits:** If possible, aim for your side or rear rather than your knees or wrists.
4. **Protect Your Head:** Use your arms to shield your head if falling forward.
5. **Get Up Slowly:** Check for injuries before standing.

Inspirational Story:

Patricia, 67, credits a fall prevention class for saving her from a serious injury. "When I slipped on some ice, my instincts kicked in, and I rolled like a pro," she says. "The neighbors thought I was doing gymnastics!"

5 Tips for Mental and Physical Resilience

Falling isn't just a physical challenge, it can also shake your confidence. Building resilience helps you bounce back emotionally and keep moving forward.

Tips for Confidence Building:

1. **Practice Self-Compassion:** Everyone falls, don't beat yourself up. I still do.
2. **Stay Active:** Regular exercise strengthens your body and boosts confidence.
3. **Learn from Mistakes:** Identify the cause of a fall and take steps to prevent it.
4. **Stay Positive:** Focus on what you can do, not what went wrong.
5. **Ask for Help:** There's no shame in using assistive devices or leaning on a friend.

Inspirational Story:
After recovering from a fall, Helen joined a Tai chi class to rebuild her confidence. "The slow, flowing movements feel like a dance," she says. "And the best part? No one cares if you wobble!"

Weekly Checklist: The Balance Challenge

Here's your 5-step challenge for improving balance and resilience this week:

1. **Try One New Exercise:** Pick a balance exercise from the list and practice it daily.
2. **Declutter Your Space:** Remove tripping hazards like loose rugs and cords.
3. **Mind Your Shoes:** Wear supportive, non-slip footwear around the house.
4. **Practice Awareness:** Pay attention to your surroundings to avoid surprises.
5. **Celebrate Progress:** Treat yourself to something fun after completing the challenge—like a dance session in your living room!

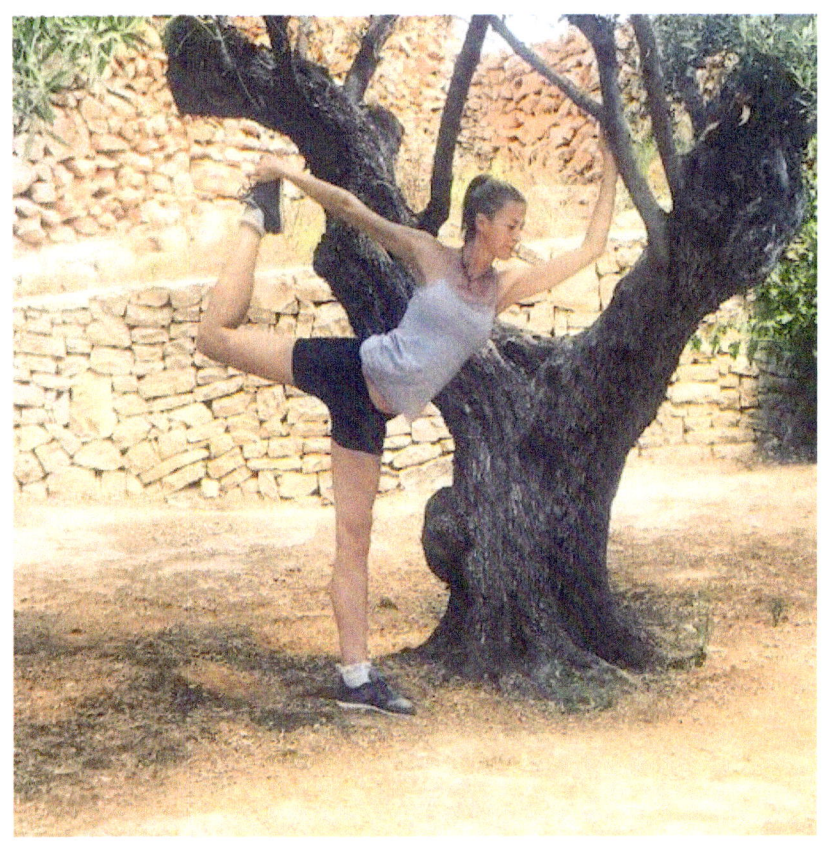

Be with the tree grounded in nature

Conclusion: Staying Grounded (Literally and Figuratively)

Balance isn't just about staying upright, it's about feeling grounded in every sense of the word. By practicing balance exercises, learning how to fall safely, and building resilience, you're not just reducing risks, you're gaining confidence and grace.

Final Humorous Anecdote:

After completing her first week of balance exercises, Margaret declared, "I'm not saying I could join the circus, but I did manage to carry a coffee cup across the room without spilling it. Progress!"

Remember, it's not about avoiding every fall, it's about rising gracefully when life gives you a nudge. With practice, humor, and a dash of determination, you'll stay steady and strong, no matter what. As my physio used to say, if it isn't broken just back up and keep walking, the body does not like to sit around.

Food, Glorious Food! Eating for Energy and Vitality

Welcome to the delicious world of eating for energy, health, and vitality! At 60 and beyond, food is more than fuel; it's a gateway to feeling amazing, staying active, and enjoying life to the fullest. This chapter is a culinary journey sprinkled with practical nutrition tips, the joy of occasional indulgence, and a big dash of humor to keep things light.

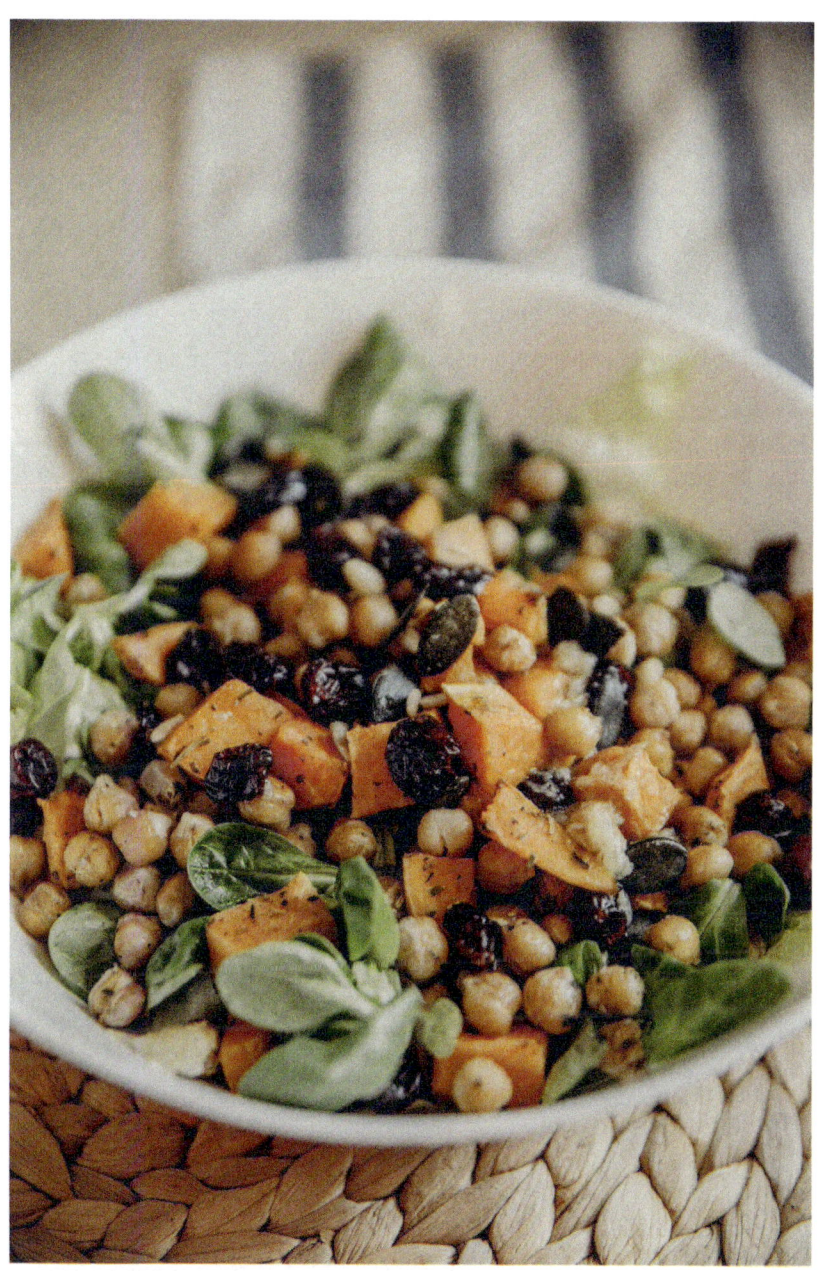

A healthy poke bowl lunch

Food is life, literally! It's the magic that powers every step, stretch, and laugh. At 60+, our nutritional needs evolve, but the joy of eating should never fade. This chapter is about fueling your body to thrive while keeping the delight alive. This is one of the most important chapters in my book. We are what we eat, how we think, react, sleep, and exercise. Oh and don't forget the aging process, a healthy balance of all the good things will help our flexibility, moods, and joy in life.

I want to bust some common myths, simplify healthy eating, and, yes, carve out space for a cheeky treat now and then, and I love my treats, I want to do it all with no cravings, which is far worse on your mind, then the temptation will creep in. You will quickly realize the only secret lie is to your subconscious; my son calls the little naughty devil in my head!. Remember, it's not about deprivation, it's about liberation through nourishment!

The Foundations of Eating for Energy

1. **Protein: The Building Blocks of Strength** Protein becomes essential for maintaining muscle mass as we age. Think lean meats, beans, tofu, and nuts. Imagine your muscles throwing a party every time you enjoy a protein-packed meal. *Tip:* Keep it playful. Name your post-workout smoothie or juice "The Muscle Maker" or "Protein Punch" to make nutrition fun!

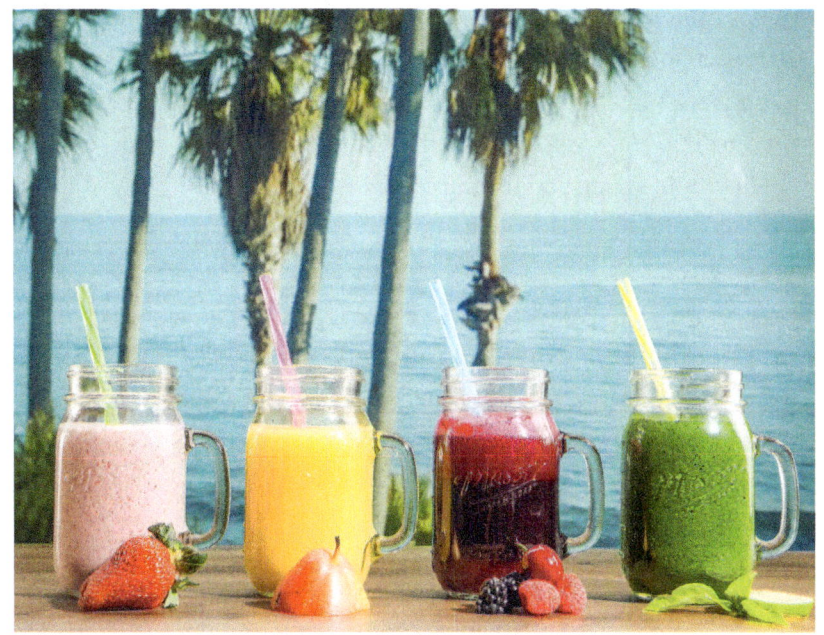

What's Your Favorite?

1.
2. **Healthy Fats: Friends, Not Foes** Avocados, olive oil, and nuts are your allies, this is contrary to all the bad press they are getting lately calories versus good health. Always think balance and a little of what you do well is the best way to go. Remember journalists must find new content every month to write about to please their editor's deadline, don't be taken in by the latest offering in a magazine. Avocados are like the little black dress of food, timeless, elegant, and always in style. Say goodbye to fearing fat and hello to glowing skin and happy joints. *Anecdote:* My friend started calling avocados "green gold." She's not wrong—they're priceless for energy and vitality.

1. **Complex Carbs: The Slow-Burn Energy Source** Whole grains, sweet potatoes, and legumes keep you energized without the sugar crash. Think of these as the kindling that keeps your internal fire burning. *Humor:* Think of white bread as a bad date—enticing at first but leaving you feeling empty.

1. **Vitamins and Minerals: Your Internal Spark Plugs** Calcium, magnesium, and vitamin D help to keep bones strong and energy levels high. Add leafy greens, dairy, and a sprinkle of sunlight to your daily routine. *Tip:* Picture yourself as a flourishing garden, water it, feed it, and bask in the sunshine!

Why Nutrition Matters Now More Than Ever

As we age, our nutritional needs shift. It's not about eating less; it's about eating smarter. Think of your plate as a palette colorful, vibrant, and filled with life. Eating well at this stage can:

- Boost energy levels.
- Support strong bones and joints.
- Improve digestion.
- Enhance mental clarity.
- Keep your heart healthy and spirits high.

If your younger self could eat pizza at midnight and wake up unscathed, your older self deserves better fuel to keep that pep in your step.

5 Top Healthy Nutritional Tips

Tip #1: Build a Balanced Plate
A balanced plate is like a symphony, with all the food groups harmonizing beautifully. Here's the cheat sheet:

- **Half Your Plate:** Fruits and veggies. Think spinach, berries, and a sprinkle of nuts.
- **One-Quarter:** Lean protein. Chicken, Turkey, fish, beans, or eggs.
- **One-Quarter:** Whole grains. Quinoa, brown rice, or whole-grain bread.
- **Bonus:** A small portion of healthy fats like avocado or olive oil.

Anecdote: The Case of the Kale Catastrophe
Jacky, a friend of mine, tried kale for the first time because "It's good for you!" She roasted it, salted it, and even doused it in olive oil. But when she bit into the first leaf, she declared, "If health tastes like this, I'd rather stay sick." Moral of the story? If you're new to superfoods, start small or find creative recipes that make them delicious, such as adding mixed seeds like sesame or chia for an explosive nutty flavor that's my favorite and the only way I can get my husband to eat kale. He thinks it is like crispy seaweed he enjoys on a Chinese meal! —Kale chips, anyone?

Tip #2: Stay Hydrated (Yes, Coffee Counts)
Hydration is a game-changer. As we age, our sense of thirst can dull. Aim for 8 glasses of water a day, add lemon or cucumber slices for flavor. And yes, coffee and tea count, but try to avoid sugary drinks. Although I find tea and coffee make me pee too much, I will stick to water after my morning coffee mixed with a few mugs of tea whilst working on my writing. However, I love the occasional wine when not writing as it makes me too sleepy and lose my sharp head. Wine is great for social

events and, though delightful, is best enjoyed in moderation!

Fun Task: Water With a Twist

Create a week's worth of spa-inspired water. Try combinations like:

- Mint and lime.
- Strawberry and basil.
- Orange and rosemary.

Snap a photo of your fanciest concoction and share it with your friends. Who says hydration can't be glamorous?

Tip #3: Embrace Protein

Protein helps maintain muscle mass and keeps you full longer. Aim to include it in every meal. Think beyond meat:

- Greek yogurt for breakfast.
- A handful of almonds as a snack.
- Lentil soup for lunch.
- Grilled salmon for dinner.

Inspirational Story: Sheila's Protein Power

Sheila added a boiled egg to her breakfast and switched to protein-rich snacks like hummus and veggies. In just a month, she felt stronger during her walks and even beat her grandson in an arm-wrestling match. Coincidence? We think not.

Tip #4: The Joy of Cheat Days

Yes, you can have your cake and eat it too, just not every day. Cheat days are about savoring life without guilt. I am so lucky that my local post walk/jog cafe on Saturdays makes delicious fat-free and low-sugar fruit cake for all the runners from the Park Run held in my park. A fab way to start your 5km from zero to walking to jogging to run. Coffee is treated immediately afterward as a reward. Plan a treat once a week:

- Ice cream with grandkids.
- A buttery croissant with coffee.
- Pizza night with friends.
- Coffee and cake after ParkRun with friends or your park aim for one hour.

Anecdote: The Chocolate Escape
One Sunday, I decided to treat myself to a chocolate bar. Before I knew it, the wrapper was empty, and my cat Sky was chasing it around the floor. Lesson learned? Indulge, but enjoy it slowly, you'll appreciate it more, and your cat won't judge you!

Tip #5: Keep It Simple
Healthy eating doesn't have to be complicated. Stick to these basics:

- **Eat Real Food:** Less processed (avoid totally if possible, check labels before buying and less takeouts unless you know they are cooked from healthy-minded kitchens, go more fresh whenever you can. Do not be afraid to ask what is in it.
- **Shop the Perimeter:** That's where the fresh produce, meat, and dairy are.
- **Meal Prep:** Plan your meals for the week to avoid last-minute unhealthy choices.

Fun Task: One-Pan Wonders
Experiment with one-pan meals. Toss chicken, veggies, and olive oil onto a baking tray. Add herbs, roast, and voila! Minimal cleanup,

maximum flavor. To be honest this is me nearly all the time. First because of my daily scheduled time and also I want to make sure I have had all the good stuff added daily so why do less a throw-in meal in one pan is my favorite way to go.

I also cook three-day meals. Day 1 is the first meal, and day 2 is the base pan now with added ingredients with more spice and rice. Day 3 I have already frozen two portions from day 1 to enjoy in a week. I often eat from the freezer. This way I know what's in it and the meal contains all the best ingredients for my fit lifestyle on the go.

Inspirational Quote
"Food is the most primitive form of comfort." – Sheilah Graham
Let's make that comfort nourishing, too.

Your Weekly Nutritional Challenge

1. **Try a new fruit or veggie every day.**
2. **Swap one processed snack for a whole-food alternative.**
3. **Hydrate—track your water intake and aim for 8 glasses.**
4. **Plan and cook one healthy meal for the week.**
5. **Schedule a guilt-free cheat day.**

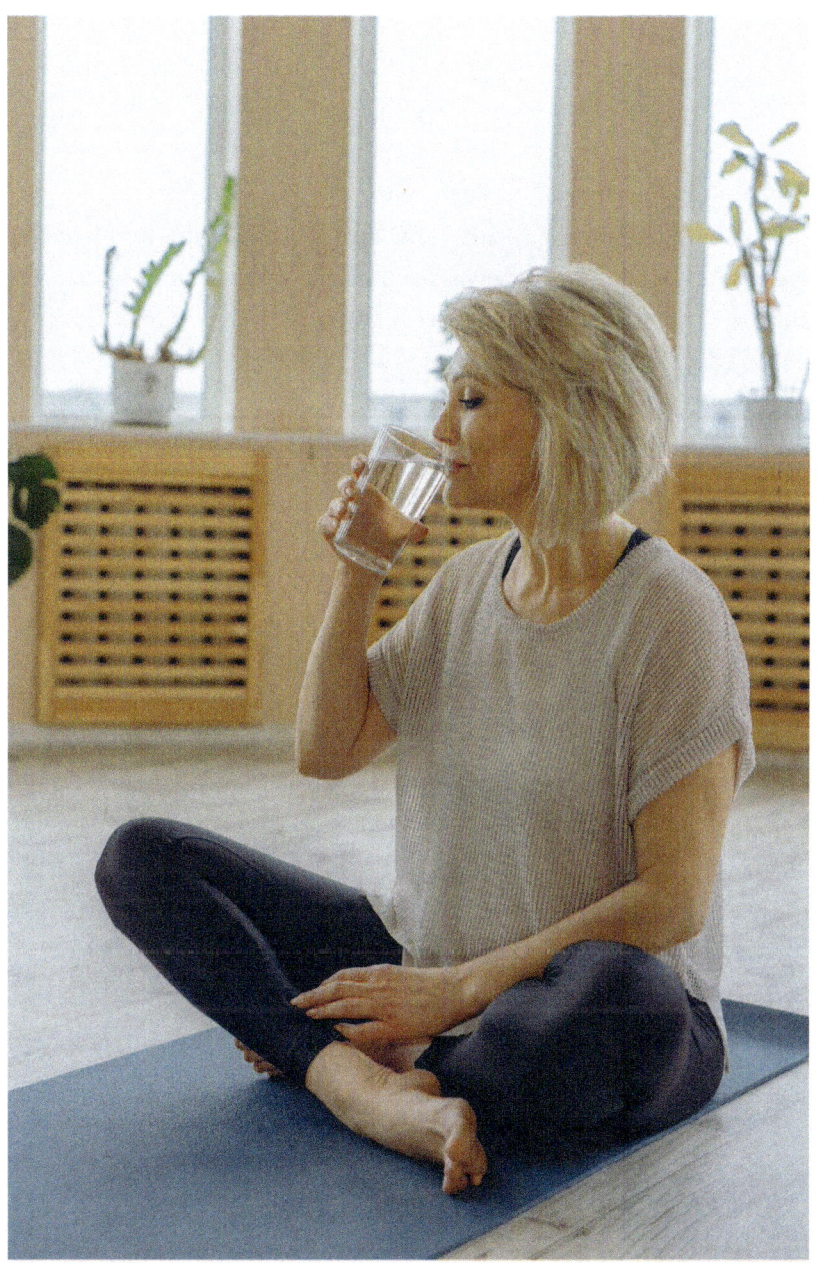

Drink plenty of filtered water is an essential part of fitness

Reminder: Progress, Not Perfection

Changing habits takes time. Celebrate the small wins and laugh at the slip-ups. Whether you're mastering kale or savoring chocolate, it's all part of the delicious journey to vitality.

The Joy (and Mischief) of Cheat Days

Who said healthy eating has to be all spinach and no cake? Cheat days are like a mini vacation for your taste buds. Plan them, savor them, and let go of any guilt. You may find that when you do, your taste buds have evolved and you simply do not want any food that is packed with addictive sugar. I can speak personally as a chocolate and cake lover before. Now I prefer homemade cakes; if I join friends for a post-exercise cafe visit, with less sugar and foods like olives, celery, radishes, and dry nuts more appealing and salty snacks.

Anecdote: Once, I decided to make my "cheat day" coincide with my granddaughter's birthday. By the end of it, we were covered in frosting and laughing like schoolgirls.

Five Tips for Simplifying Healthy Eating

1. **Plan, Don't Panic** A weekly meal plan can make shopping and cooking a breeze. Bonus: fewer impulse buys!
2. **Batch Cooking for the Win** Make soups, stews, or roasted veggies in large quantities. Freeze portions for those days you don't feel like cooking.
3. **Hydrate Like a Pro** Water is your secret weapon. Feeling sluggish? Sip some H2O. I highly recommend a water filter system to avoid

all the new chemicals being added to our water, I would not be without mine. My local bar even has a mains water filtration system for table water. Need a glow-up? Water again. *Humor:* Who knew the fountain of youth was sitting in your kitchen?
4. **Keep Snacks Handy** Nuts (not too many high in calories, I love them too), celery, olives, radishes chopped ready in the fridge, hummus with added fresh herbs such as cilantro, fruit, or a hard-boiled egg can be lifesavers when hunger strikes. Avoid those "hanger" moments!
5. **Ditch the Diet Mentality** Focus on what you *can* eat rather than what you can't. Healthy eating is about abundance, not restriction.

Inspirational Stories: Real Women, Real Results

- ***Shona's Journey*:** At 65 starting out as a beginner with me in Spain for 10 days before returning home to kick-start her new regime of fitness. Shona transformed her health by swapping sugary breakfasts for smoothies packed with greens and protein. Her energy levels soared, and she even started a Zumba class! Try it, it works for me.
- ***Linda's Late-Night Revelation*:** Linda learned that her evening snack of yogurt with honey was perfect for curbing cravings and aiding sleep.

Lighthearted Food Challenges:

- **The Rainbow Plate Challenge:** Eat five different colors in one meal.
- **DIY Healthy Pizza Night**: Use whole-grain crusts, load up on

veggies, and indulge in a sprinkle of cheese.
- **Water Drinking Game**: Every time you check your phone, take a sip of filtered water. Hydration and screen breaks? Genius!

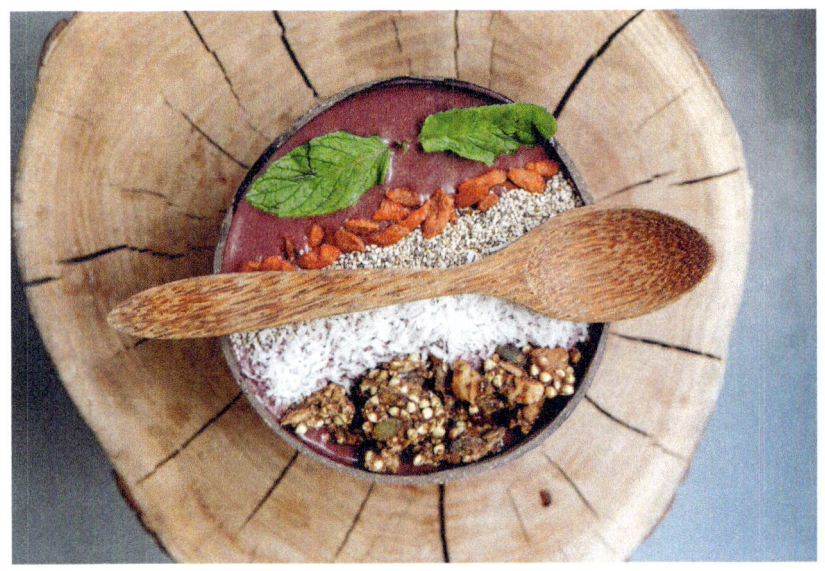

You eat with your eyes first, make your dishes colorful

Conclusion: Savour the Journey

Food is more than fuel, it's an experience, a connection, and a joy. By embracing balance and adding a dash of humor to your plate, you'll nourish not just your body but your spirit, too. So go ahead, stretch the truth a little on your cheat days, but always eat for vitality.

I cannot begin to tell you how important healthy food and water intake can completely change how you feel, your energy levels, your moods regardless of what's happening in your life and simply that grin and glow that people ask what are you on I want to bottle it, why do you never appear to get tired or age much?

And remember: Every bite is a chance to fuel your fabulousness!

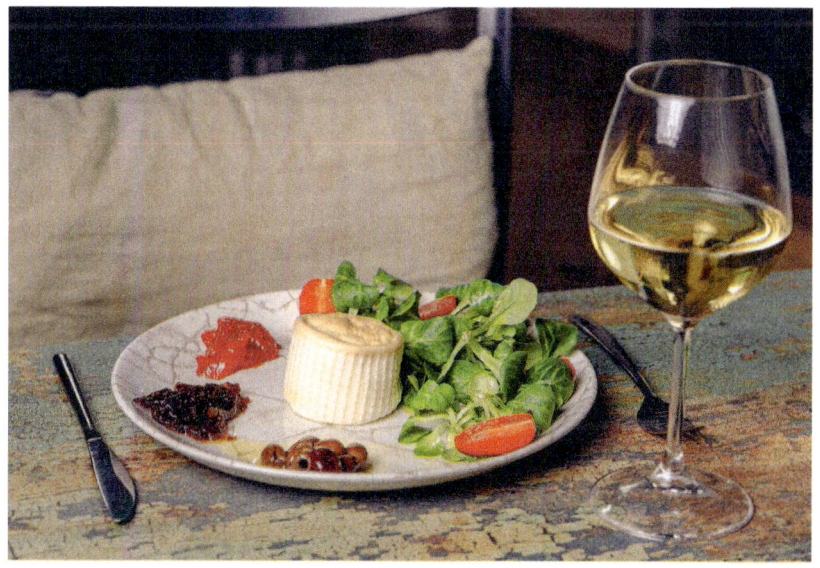

You Deserve It

A cheeky vino on cheat days is even better. Enjoy.

Dressing the Part: Workout Gear or Glam Gear?

If the saying **"dress for success"** holds in the boardroom, why shouldn't it apply to your workouts (or even your post-yoga coffee dates)? Dressing the part isn't just about looking the part—it's about feeling ready, capable, and maybe just a little bit fabulous. Whether you're sporting neon leggings to Zumba or a sleek black tracksuit on your morning walk, the right outfit can transform your energy and confidence.

The Power of the Right Outfit

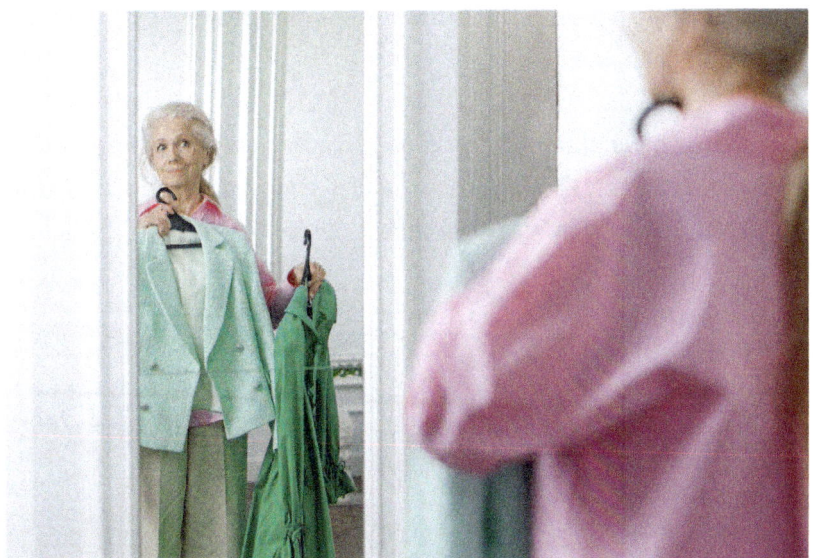

"Confidence starts with the right gear—choose what makes you feel unstoppable!"

From Lycra to the Lounge: The Evolution of Activewear

It wasn't always this glamorous, was it? Back in 70s, workout attire was synonymous with baggy sweatshirts and shiny tracksuit bottoms. Now, activewear is a billion-dollar industry offering styles to suit every personality. You can strut into a yoga class feeling like a goddess in high-waisted leggings or take your morning walk in chic trainers that could double as runway material. However, as we grow in our fitness what looked great in the shop may not be next week. Sore feet and blisters.

"Elegance is when the inside is as beautiful as the outside" - **Coco Chanel**

Fun Tip: *Want an instant energy boost? Pick workout gear in bright colors like coral, turquoise, or lime green. Studies show that vibrant colors can elevate your mood, even before you start moving!*

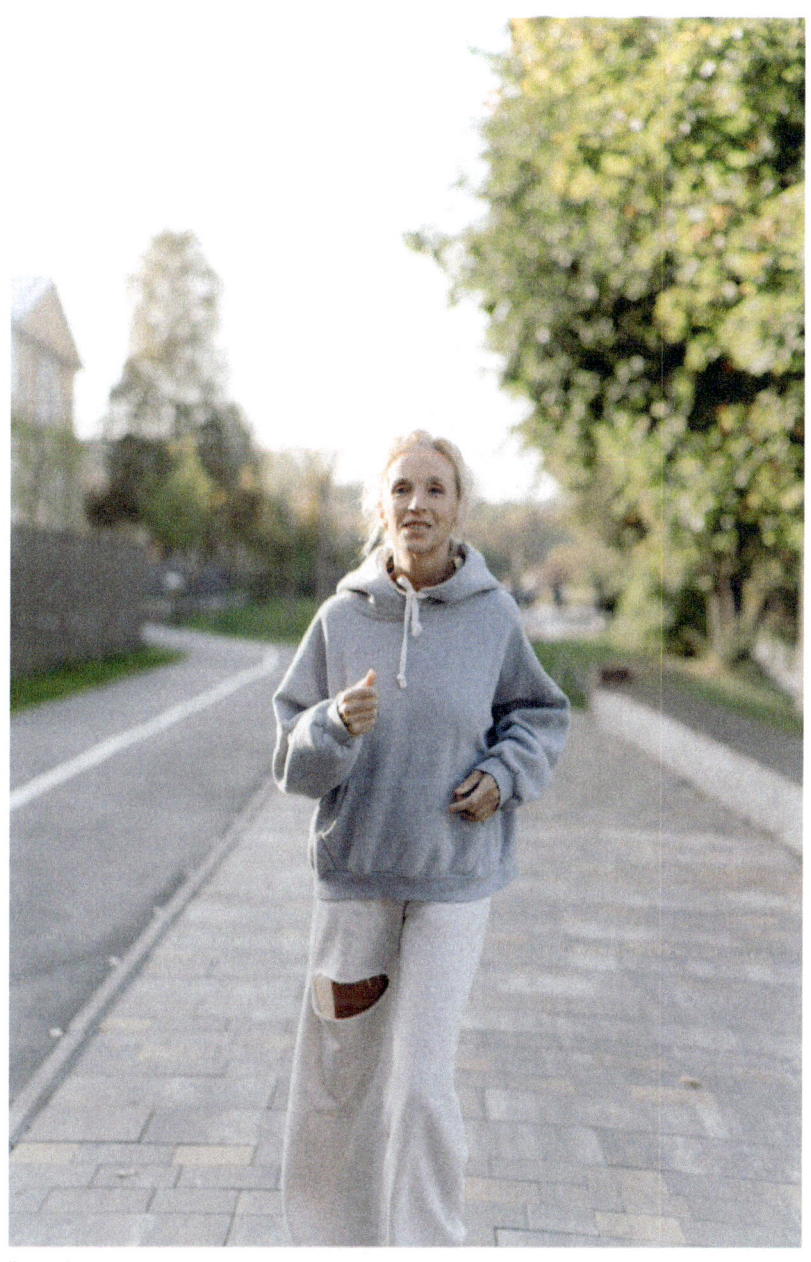

"Confidence never goes out of style—own your fitness journey, one step at a time!"
cxli

As a coordinator of my retreats for 17 years in Spain, I used to believe I had seen it all before, my guests never failed to surprise me, one with 15-year-old trainers, the shoes had gone all hard and not breathable for the warm weather for walking.

The week before my guests' retreat I would send them a 'What to bring list for their fitness holiday to suit walking, jogging, yoga, and relaxing'. I should have had shares in my local ladies' underwear and sports stores. Many of my guests did come with the kit list, but they quickly realized that their sports bras were ill-fitting or had lost all support. They had leggings that were worn out and either trainers not fit for purpose only general park walk and socks. I had become a personal shopper too!

Spain has a hot climate in summer and moderate in winter months. When it is very hot in the summer non breathable trainers or non-wick-away socks were also a serious issue. If when out exercising your body cannot breathe adequately, you can become irate or anxious or your breathing becomes labored. From my guests' experiences, it became necessary to stop and cool off. I know from my own experience of training in England to Spain it is very very different. Now I carry a mini umbrella in my backpack.

Light-Hearted Anecdote: Remember when you thought yoga pants were just for yoga? Now they're your go-to for groceries, walks, and maybe the occasional Netflix binge. Who knew spandex could be so versatile?

Fit, Function, and Fabulous: What to Look for in Workout Gear

Not all leggings are created equal, and no one wants to discover that during a deep squat. I always wear black or blue leggings. It can be common for ladies after having babies and seniors to experience a bit of urinary leakage.

My Top Tip: Always visit the powder room before the gym or any exercise to avoid any embarrassing leakage issues. If it did happen under any exertion black or blue leggings will save you until you can change!

My new guest Julie, had come to get fit and lose weight and enjoy learning how to create healthy meals. Julie assured me she would be fine and did not want to buy a new pair of suitable trainers for during and post-retreat. After a few days, I could tell she appeared to be limping. I asked what was wrong and she said I'm fine.

Another day passed and clearly, she was struggling to walk. I asked to see her feet. I had my suspicions and the blisters were worse than I could have imagined! Shock horror she needed special plasters and pharmacy care. I insisted she do some shopping to continue with her holiday. We maxed out at the sports shop to buy new shoes and wick-away socks. The result was she needed to take a day off valuable training with me, all because of the badly fitting trainers.

It was always Julie's good intention to start a fitness program one day in the future, but that was 15 years ago stored in her wardrobe she was hanging onto. I can be a very insistent Mum when I want to be and that was that training shoes and socks duly purchased!

Another Expert Tip: Always make sure you wear your new trainers by walking in them for a few days to let your feet and shoes settle together. That way they shouldn't blister and always go to a professional shop to get measured up for and then to check your gait, which is how you would walk or run to receive the correct support for you. We are all different.

The same applies to your kit: always wash it first, especially socks from new. Why even these items cause blisters too? One of my running friends, Jim, a very experienced Iron Man competitor trained all year to go to the Canary Islands to complete. He was running a half marathon and yes in new socks!!

I couldn't believe it when he told me he had made the ultimate rooky mistake of new socks that had caused serious blisters. He had to retire. He had to walk the walk of shame to all his friends and family who had traveled to the Islands to support him. An error he will never forget.

Lesson learned: Do not be so familiar to think you are experienced enough to break the basic kit rules.

What Gear to prioritize

1. **Fabric That Breathes:** Look for moisture-wicking materials that keep you cool and dry. Cotton may be comfy, but it's a sweat sponge. Especially socks.
2. **Compression:** A little snugness can do wonders for muscle support and recovery (and it doesn't hurt that it smooths things out, too!).
3. **Supportive Footwear:** Whether you're hitting the trail or dancing in your living room, shoes are very important. Seek professional store guidance when buying.
4. **Pockets or Waist Belt:** Who doesn't want a place for their keys, phone, or that emergency snack? I prefer a running belt around my waist with my water bottle.
5. **Style:** If you don't feel amazing in it, you're less likely to wear it. Find something that makes you smile!

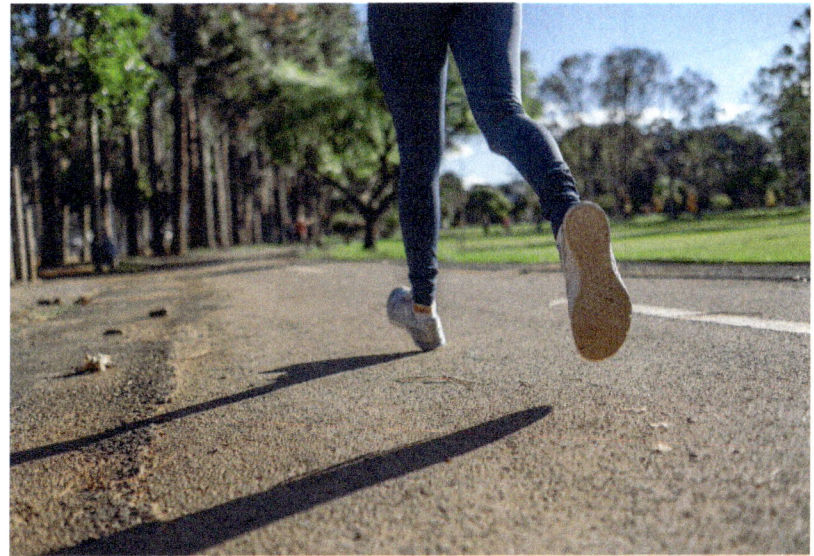

"Step into fitness with the right shoes—because every journey starts from the ground up!"

Glam Wear: Transforming Your Look After the Gym

One of the best parts about modern workout gear? It doubles as casual glam wear. Throw on a flowing cardigan, and a statement necklace, and voila, you're ready for lunch with friends. Easy fix for me in my backpack.

Quick Glam Checklist:
- Swap trainers for ankle boots.
- Add a lightweight scarf for flair or buff for the neck. I wouldn't be without mine.
- Keep a compact makeup kit in your bag (a swipe of lipstick works wonders!).

Inspirational Story: Meet Clara, 62, who found her confidence by upgrading her gym wardrobe. "I used to hide in oversized T-shirts," she laughs, "but then I bought a pair of hot-pink leggings, and suddenly I felt unstoppable. Now, I'm not just walking faster, I'm walking taller!"

Dressing for Every Season

Staying active means braving all kinds of weather, so let's talk layering:

- **Winter:** Thermal leggings, a cozy fleece, a warm buff and hat, and a windproof jacket. Don't forget gloves!
- **Spring:** Lightweight layers you can peel off as you warm up. Baseball cap.
- **Summer:** Breathable shorts or leggings with a moisture-wicking crop top.
- **Autumn:** Think long sleeves and leggings with reflective details for shorter days.

Humorous Interjection: "Layers are like friends: you want them close, but not too clingy. If your jacket is suffocating you mid-run, it's time to upgrade."

Common Wardrobe Mishaps (and How to Avoid Them)

- **The See-Through Leggings Surprise:** Always check your leggings in natural light before wearing them out and see-through yoga pants too!
- **The Trainer Squeak:** A baby powder can save your soles (and sanity).

- **The Wardrobe Malfunction:** Test your outfit with a few stretches and squats at home. If it shifts too much, it's not gym-ready.

Budget-Friendly Tips for Fabulous Fitness Fashion

1. **Shop Sales:** End-of-season sales can be a goldmine.
2. **Thrift Stores:** Sometimes, people donate brand-new gear.
3. **Online Marketplaces:** Search for lightly used or discounted items.
4. **Mix High and Low:** Splurge on the essentials (like shoes) and save on accessories.

Fun Task: Challenge yourself to build a complete workout outfit for under $50. Bonus points if it makes you feel like a rock star!

Call to Action: Your Fitness Wardrobe Makeover

Take a look at your current workout wardrobe. Is it inspiring you? If not, treat yourself to a few pieces that make you feel amazing. Because here's the truth: when you look good, you feel good and when you feel good, you move more.

My Top Tip: All lycra-type leggings, crop tops, and jogging socks must be washed by hand and hung to drip dry in the shower immediately post-training session. I always bring my kit into the shower as soon as I get home.

I have a watered-down version of normal hand soap and wash gear in the shower. It is then hung on a removable rack I hook over the glass door. Usually, overnight my kit is ready to wear, and if not in the winter I have two sets of fitness gear.

The main reason is apart from the fact quality branded kit can be very expensive, also the washing machine action can spin the life out of your kit very quickly and it can begin to go baggy having lost its integrity. Fabric conditioners will quickly spoil the elastic part of the lycra, ruining it fast in my personal experience, to lose its integrity. Never tumble dry your kit either. The same fast destroying applies. I don't like shopping very much or have the time. I would rather take good care of my kit aside from the cost.

Conclusion: It's Not Just Clothes, It's Confidence

Whether you're hitting the gym, the trail, or just the couch after a well-deserved rest day, what you wear can set the tone for how you feel. So, embrace your style, experiment with colors, and remember: the most important thing you can wear is confidence.

"You're never too old to wear neon—and you're certainly never too old to rock it.

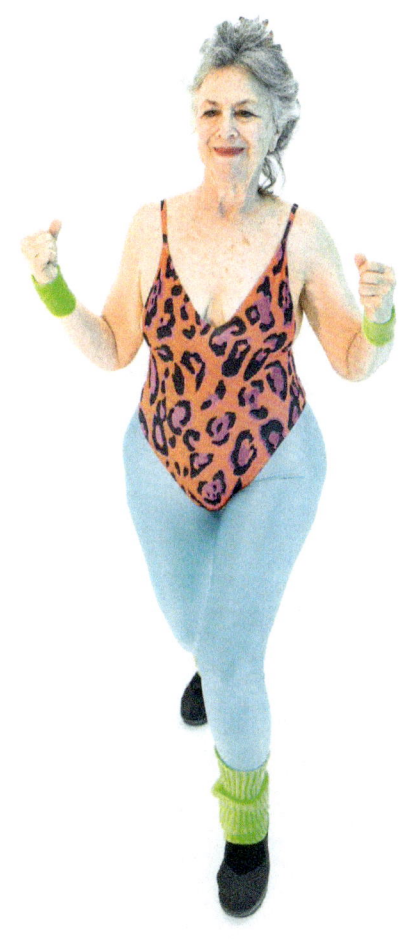

Wear what makes you feel great and confident

cl

Workout Buddies: From Friends to Furry Companions

Who needs a personal trainer when you have a furry friend eagerly waiting by the door with a leash in their mouth? Dogs are the ultimate fitness companions, always ready for a walk, never judging your pace, and making every outing an adventure. Even if you don't own a dog, the joys of walking a four-legged friend can transform your fitness journey.

In this chapter, we'll explore how furry friends can inspire healthier habits, the benefits of walking for you and your dog, and how you can even get paid to walk.

"Walking a dog burns calories, builds muscle, and occasionally earns you a new best friend at the park."

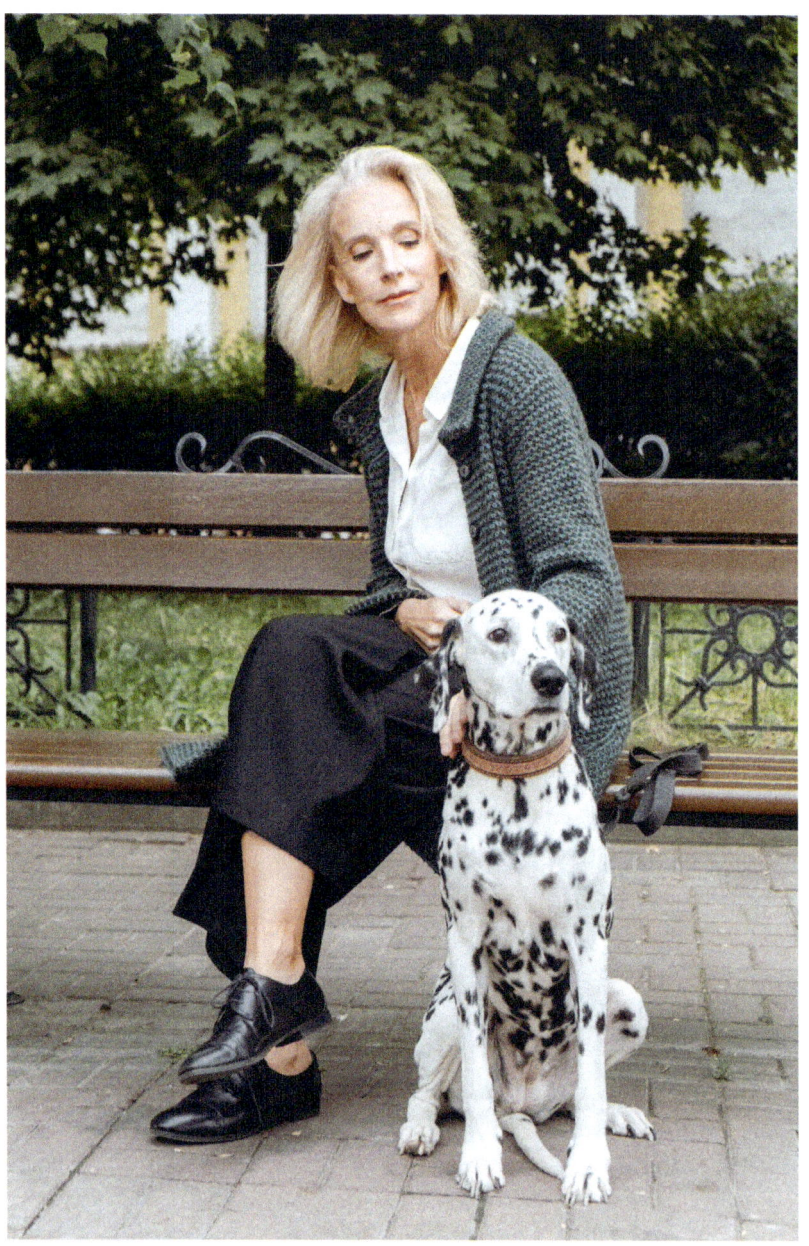

"Fitness is better with a furry friend—because every step is more fun with a wagging tail!"

Pets have a magical way of making life brighter, they're not just adorable companions; they're fitness motivators in disguise.

Whether it's the boundless energy of a dog, the playful curiosity of a cat, or even the serene pace of a tortoise, furry (or feathered, or scaly) friends have a knack for keeping you active, engaged, and smiling. Here's Athena bouncing along packed with high energy to keep any walker/jogger fit.

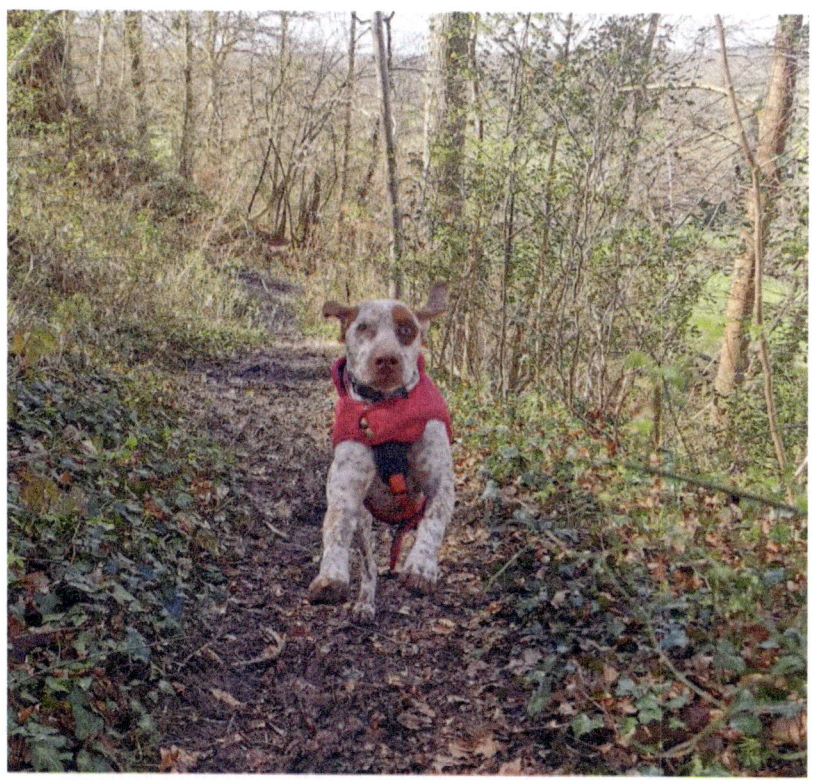

"Unleash the joy—because fitness feels like freedom when you're running wild with your best friend!"

The Fitness Benefits of Pets

Walks with Purpose

A dog's wagging tail is nature's perfect personal trainer. Rain or shine, they'll remind you it's time to move. And let's be honest, who can resist that "take me outside" face?

Pro Tip: Turn your walks into mini adventures by exploring new trails or parks together.

Playtime Equals Cardio:

Whether it's tossing a ball, playing tug-of-war, or chasing a laser pointer, pet playtime is an excellent way to sneak in some heart-healthy activity. Bonus: your pet gets their workout, too!

Stress Reduction on Four Legs:

Studies show that petting an animal lowers blood pressure and reduces stress. Pair that with some gentle stretching or yoga, and you've got a wellness routine built around furry snuggles.

Furry Friends with Fitness Perks

Dogs: The ultimate accountability partners, dogs thrive on routine and will happily drag you outside for daily walks, hikes, or even runs.

Cats: While less enthusiastic about fitness, cats love interactive toys that can get you moving, like feather wands or laser pointers. Plus, they're great yoga companions—ever tried Downward Dog with a curious cat underfoot?

Small Pets: Rabbits, ferrets, and guinea pigs may not join you for a jog, but their playful antics can inspire impromptu movement.

Birds: Encourage them to flap their wings by moving with them.

Dance party, anyone?

Turtles and Tortoises: These slower companions remind you to embrace mindfulness and enjoy the journey rather than rush through it.

Funny Fitness Moments with Pets

The Unplanned Sprint

Ever had a dog take off after a squirrel? Congratulations, you've just completed a surprise 100-meter dash!

Yoga Interrupted

Pets love to join yoga sessions—usually by sprawling on your mat, pawing at your hair, or licking your face during Warrior Pose.

All my cats adore yoga class music and mats. In Spain, we always have our classes on the beach or pool terrace. In no time the cats, who had been chilling somewhere would hear the music starting and the mats rolled out. A guest called Sophie said whilst she'd enjoyed the pool terrace class she didn't get a cat sitting on her like the other guests. I had 12 rescue cats then, but only 6 were interested in sitting on my guests or taking over their mats. Sometimes I would have to let my cats have their mats. It was adorable and slightly chaotic, usually resulting in photo sessions for them to take home. Isabelle is now sixteen. Cats love Yoga!

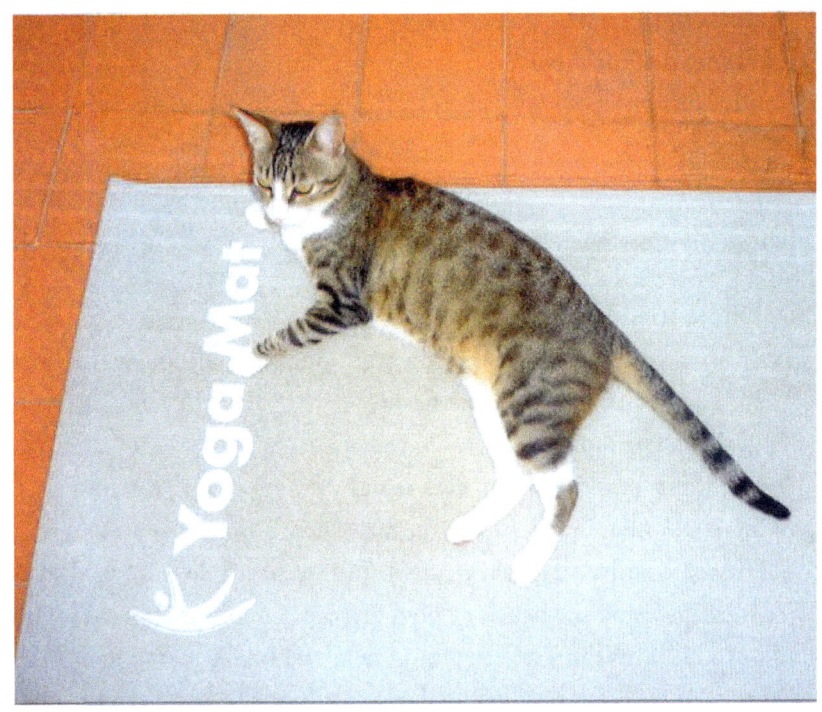

"Find your zen—even if your yoga buddy prefers the 'purrfect' pose of total relaxation!"

Fetch Gone Wrong:

Sometimes the ball doesn't come back—or worse, your dog decides to run off with it, initiating a hilarious game of chase.

My Cat's Choice Workout:

A cat sitting on your lap during stretches? That's resistance training.

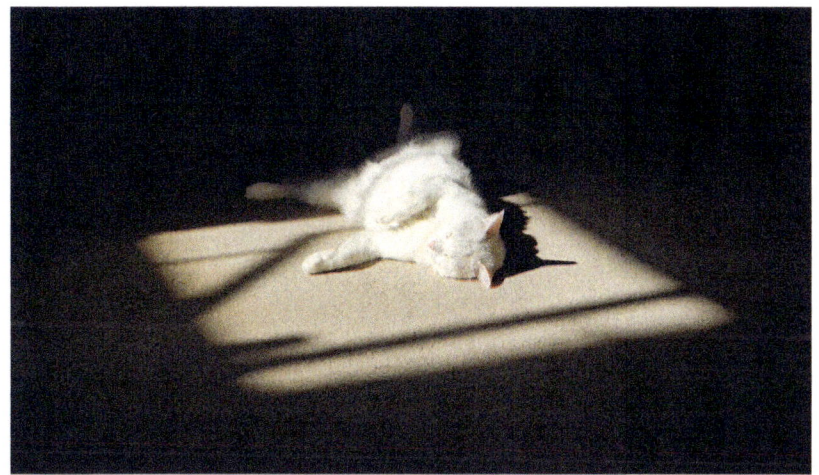

"Master the art of the ultimate savasana—this yoga guru knows how to truly relax!"

Sky just can't be bothered

Creating a Fitness Routine with Your Pet

Structured Walks. Dogs love routine, so aim for regular morning or evening walks. Add some variety with short jogging intervals or outdoor games.

Interactive Play:
Use toys, balls, or homemade contraptions to engage your pet while you stay active. A simple game of fetch or chase can double as your daily cardio.

Training Together:
Teaching your dog new tricks or practicing obedience commands isn't just good for them, it's mentally stimulating for you, too.

Doga (Dog Yoga) Even Goat Yoga:
Yes, it's a thing! Practice stretches with your dog beside you, or gently

involve them in poses. If nothing else, it's a guaranteed giggle session. With goats, they roam around the dwarf type, look on the internet for funny goat yoga videos.

Adventures Beyond the Backyard:

Hikes and Trails: Dogs make excellent hiking companions. Pack water for both of you and hit the trails for a dose of nature and exercise. If you are training by yourself you have your little bodyguard and buddy.

Dog Parks: A chance for socializing for both you and your dog! Join in the fun by jogging alongside them or tossing toys.

Swimming: If your pet loves water, consider a swim session. It's a low-impact exercise for both of you and a perfect way to cool off on hot days.

The Emotional Benefits of Pet-Assisted Fitness

- **Unconditional Encouragement**
- **Pets don't care if you're sweating or stumbling—they're just thrilled to be by your side.**
- **Companionship, you can chat along too and never interrupt back.**
- **Having a furry friend along for the journey makes every walk, stretch, or play session feel like an adventure shared.**
- **Mindful Movement**
- **Pets live in the moment, and their joy can remind you to slow down and savor the simple pleasures of moving your body.**

For Pet-Free Readers: Borrow the Joy

Don't have a pet? No problem! Volunteer at a shelter, offer to walk a friend's dog or visit a local cat café. It's a wonderful way to experience the benefits of animal companionship without long-term commitments.

Heartwarming Stories

Pet-Fueled Fitness Inspiration

Linda and Max, aged 65. Linda never considered herself a runner until Max, her energetic Labrador, came into her life. Now, they tackle 5Ks together, Max grinning all the way and Linda feeling fitter than ever.

Carol and Mittens, Aged 70

Carol's cat Mittens loves to join her yoga sessions. Carol swears Mittens purrs louder during meditation, making every session twice as relaxing.

Coleen and Bella, aged 68

Coleen's rescued Bichon Frise Bella helped him discover the joy of long walks. Together, they've explored local parks, and beaches, and even tackled a few gentle hiking trails, and taken holidays and weekends away.

I hear you saying but I do not have a dog and it is not possible for me to keep a dog. What is the solution?

Do not worry. This is what I do to help myself to get fit and that of a dog belonging to someone who for whatever reason is unable to take it for a regular walk, maybe an elderly person or a disabled owner. You will become super fit without thinking it is keeping fit in the chore sense every week. You will love to go out with a sense of purpose. It is a great distraction. Fit you and fit your dog in no time!

Why not let someone else's dog pay for your workout? These days, there are countless websites where you can sign up to be a dog walker and earn money while you stroll. Imagine it: you're getting your steps in, bonding with a furry friend, and getting paid for it all without the vet bills or chewed-up shoes. It's like having a personal trainer with paws and a wagging tail, except they won't yell at you to do burpees. Plus, the more enthusiastic the dog, the better your cardio. Who knew fitness could be so profitable and adorable?

Why Walking is a (Paw-some) Exercise:

Walking is a low-impact, accessible form of exercise with big benefits, especially when you add a dog to the mix. It's great for your heart, your mood, and your social life. Works for me even as a runner. Now I have a very fit Frenchie to walk/run with, he always beats me up the hills, and we compete with each other for sure.

Top Benefits of Walking with Dogs

1. **Heart Health:** Walking strengthens your cardiovascular system and reduces blood pressure.
2. **Mood Booster:** Spending time with dogs releases feel-good hormones like serotonin.
3. **Consistent Motivation:** Dogs don't take no for an answer when it's walk time!
4. **Social Opportunities:** Dogs are natural icebreakers and make meeting new people easier.
5. **Double the Fun:** You get fit, and so does your furry companion.

Inspirational Story:

My daughter Sunny, a professional dog walker, rescued a beautiful French Pointer from the pound and as soon as Athena was old enough started walking her on the beach. Sunny "At first, I thought I was doing it for her," she says. "But now I realize he's been helping me just as much, I've lost weight, feel more energetic and fitter, and made friends with half the neighborhood!"

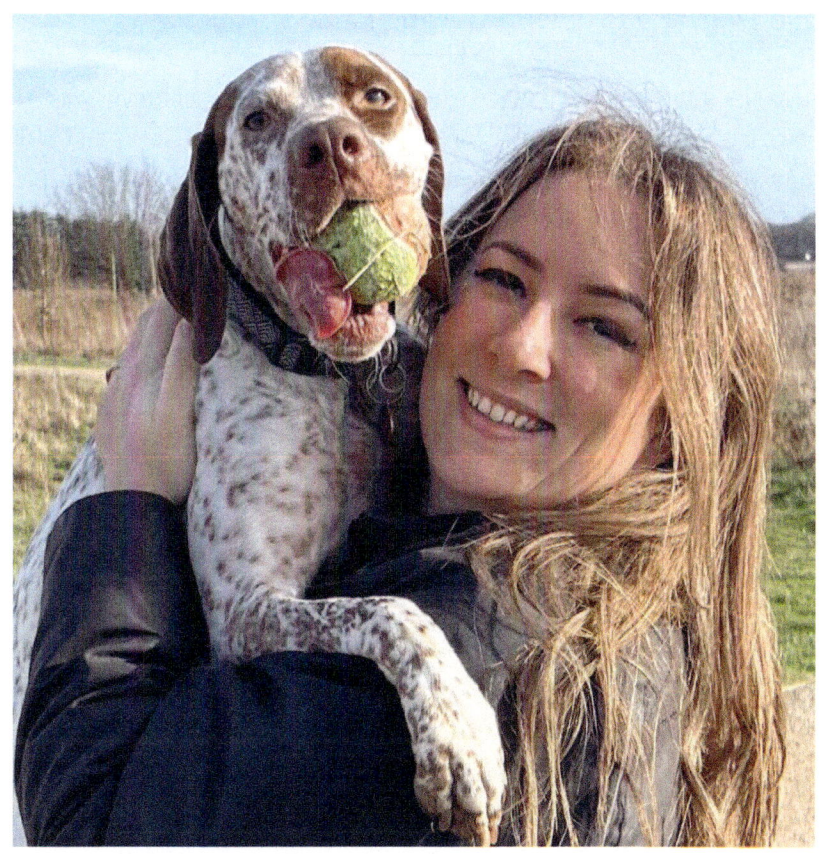

"Sunny and her loyal partner Athena prove that fitness and furry friends can be a rewarding profession—and a whole lot of love!"

Fun Task:

Set a goal to walk at least 15 minutes a day with your dog or a borrowed one. Keep track of how you feel after each walk. Take your dog to a local Saturday ParkRun with all the others with dogs on leads. They do enjoy every minute of a few hundred people both running and walking. It's very nicely exciting for them.

No Dog? No Problem! Getting Paid to Walk

If you are not already a dog owner, why not walk someone else's and earn cash while you're at it? Dog-walking platforms like Rover and Wag connect you with local pet owners, turning exercise into a side hustle.

Steps to Get Started:

1. **Sign Up on a Dog-Walking Platform:** Create a profile showcasing your love for dogs.
2. **Set Your Schedule:** Choose times that work best for you.
3. **Meet the Pups:** Arrange a meet-and-greet to ensure compatibility.
4. **Start Walking:** Enjoy the health benefits and a little extra income.
5. **Build Relationships:** Regular clients mean more walks and furry friendships.

I am a paid dog walker in my spare time for owners who are either too old or have had accidents to take their dogs for weekly walks. What a great way to combine your fitness and be paid three times a week for an hour each time. The best bit is no food to buy, vet bills, or dirty dogs to wash. I have 5 indoor cats. It's not possible for me with my schedule to keep a dog full-time. It is a win-win situation. There are plenty of websites to offer your services.

Just make sure you get insurance to cover yourself although some dog walking sites automatically offer insurance included.

Fun Task:

Research local dog-walking opportunities or offer to walk a friend's dog. I am a paid dog walker in my spare time for owners, who are either too old or have had accidents and unable to exercise their dogs regularly. What a great way to combine your fitness and get paid for it three times a week for an hour each time. Helping others is benefitting you too. It also is the greatest reason to go out when it's cold or raining. Your furry friend expects it.

The Fitness Power of Play

Walking is just the start, playing with dogs is a full-body workout disguised as fun. Fetch, tug-of-war, and chase games can get your heart pumping and your muscles moving.
Ways to Play for Fitness:

1. **Fetch-and-Sprint:** Throw a ball and jog alongside your dog to retrieve it.
2. **Tug-of-War Toning:** Strengthen your arms with a friendly tug session.
3. **Obstacle Courses:** Create a backyard course for you and your dog to navigate together.
4. **Park Games:** Join other dog owners for group activities like Frisbee or hide-and-seek.
5. **Water Fun:** If your dog loves swimming, play fetch in the water for a low-impact workout.

Inspirational Story:
Helen, now 61, turned her daily walks with her Golden Retriever, Daisy, into mini fitness challenges. "We added jogging intervals, uphill climbs, and even a few sprints. Daisy loves it, and I've never felt stronger!"

Humorous Anecdote:
I was asked to walk a cute dachshund called Frankie. His mum is a fitness instructor, no surprise how fast he walked in the park. He may have short legs, I laughed, but he left me in the dust with those tiny legs underneath his warm jacket moving like magic. All the work was going on underneath. A little man is always on a mission. His owner kept him

at pace, one pace fast.
Fun Task:
Plan a playful outing with your dog this weekend. Bonus points if you both end up panting happily by the end.

Dressing the Part for Doggy Workouts

Walking a dog isn't just about the leash, you also need the right gear to make your outings comfortable and enjoyable.
Essential Dog-Walking Gear:

1. **Comfortable Shoes:** Opt for sturdy, supportive walking shoes.
2. **Weather-Appropriate Clothing:** Think lightweight layers, rain jackets, or hats for sunny days. A backpack for keys, mobile, money, and tissues.
3. **Dog Accessories:** A reliable leash, poop bags, and water bottles are must-haves.
4. **Hands-Free Leashes:** Perfect for adding a jog or using your arms freely.
5. **Bright Colors or Reflective Gear:** Stay visible during early morning or evening walks.

I once forgot my raincoat during a downpour but had a spare for my doggy walking duties. "We got back to Kendall's house soaking wet, " his owner laughed. I was not only wet but had fallen over and was covered in mud down my back and bottom—but at least Kendall looked dashing in his little yellow jacket!"

Fun Task:

Create your ultimate dog-walking outfit and test it out on your next walk. Snap a picture to document your stylish fitness adventure!

Track your steps and see how much ground you can cover weekly to write in your journal.

Weekly Checklist: The Furry Fitness Challenge

Ready to embrace the joys of walking with a wagging tail? Here's your 5-step challenge:

1. **Walk Daily:** Commit to 15–30 minutes of walking each day with a dog.
2. **Mix It Up:** Add intervals of jogging or hills for an extra challenge.
3. **Play Together:** Incorporate a playful game like fetch into your routine.
4. **Track Your Progress:** Use a fitness app to log steps and distance.
5. **Connect with Others:** Join a dog-walking group or community event.

Conclusion: Four Paws and a Purpose

Dogs have an uncanny ability to inspire joy, movement, and connection. Whether you're walking your furry friend, borrowing a neighbor's, or starting a dog-walking side hustle, the rewards are immeasurable for both your body and your soul.

So, leash up, step out, and embrace the simple pleasure of walking with a furry friend. Fitness has never been so adorable or so rewarding. If you are dog walking or taking your dog it will be getting super fit too.

Your pet isn't just your companion, they're your partner in wellness. They keep you active, lift your spirits, and make every day more joyful. So whether it's a morning walk, a game of fetch, or simply stretching on the floor together, embrace the bond you share with your furry friend. It's fitness with heart, tail wags, and maybe a few extra kisses.

"Dogs Do Speak, but only to those who know how to listen." ~ **Orhan Pamuk**

Tech and Tracksuits: Embracing Fitness Gadgets

Gone are the days when fitness was just about lacing up your trainers and hitting the pavement now with tracking apps everything on your adventures can be saved for later viewing and where you have been that day to create different routes. Now, your watch can tell you everything from your heart rate to how many hours you slept (or didn't).

"**Fitness gadgets track your steps, your sleep, and your heart rate—but sadly, not how fabulous you look in your tracksuit.**"

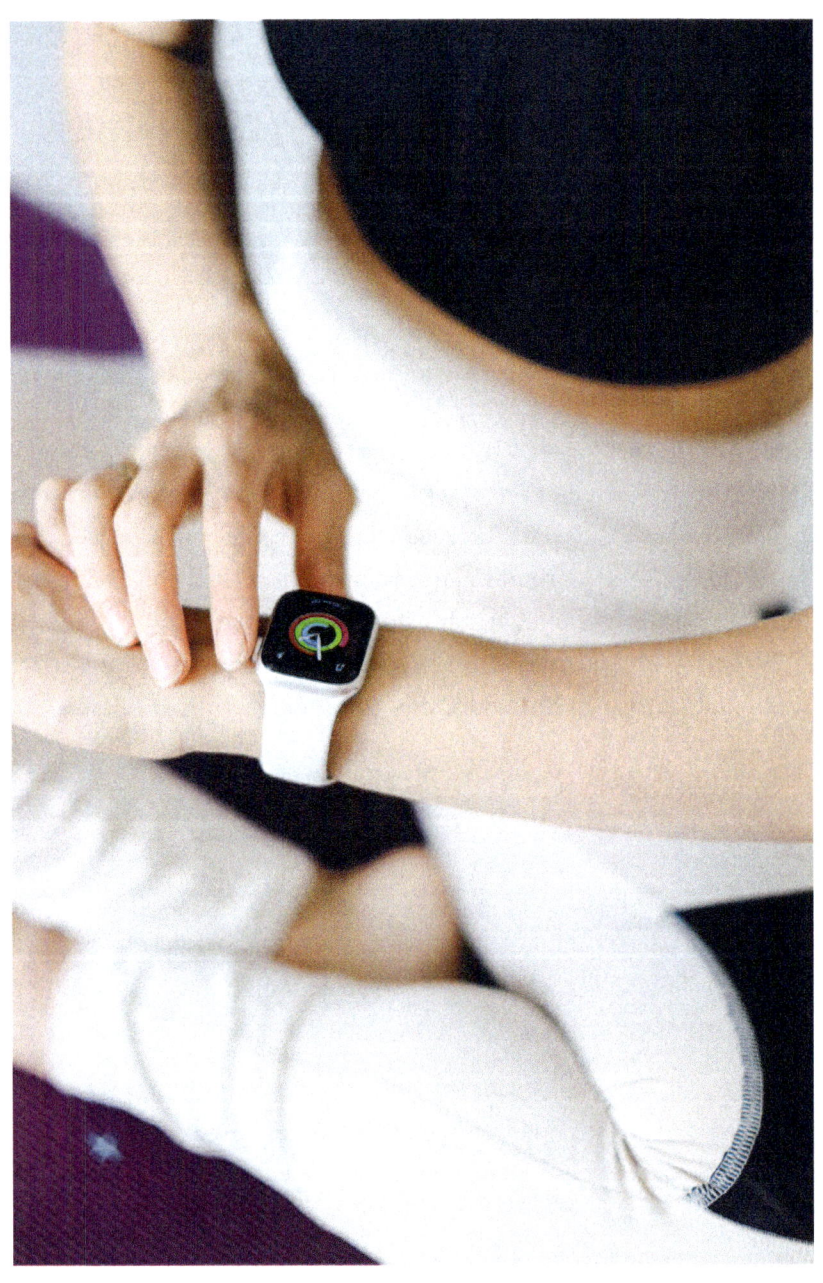

Tec Meets Fitness: Invest in a Sports Watch to Monitor Your Progress

Fitness Meets The Digital Age:

At 60, technology has brought a whole new dimension to staying active—and let's not forget the fashion revolution that transformed workout gear into something both functional and fabulous. From smartwatches to high-tech leggings, this chapter is all about embracing the intersection of tech, tracksuits, and a touch of flair.

The Gadget Debate:

Some people love their fitness gadgets; others think they're glorified pedometers. Wherever you fall, remember: The goal isn't perfection—it's progress. Use the tools that work for you, and don't stress about the rest.

The Fitness Tracker Drama:

Ever been accused by your smartwatch of "not moving enough"? There's nothing quite like having a piece of tech tell you to get off the couch—especially when you were just about to. Haha, I hear you cry out.

The Fitness App & Tec Rabbit Hole

There's an app for everything these days. Want a personal trainer? There's an app. Need someone to yell "Get moving!" to you? Also an app. Just don't spend so much time picking an app that you forget to work out. From yoga tutorials to guided walking meditations, apps offer a world of possibilities. You can choose workouts that suit your style, your pace, and your mood.

Don't like running? No problem—there's an app that tracks your progress while walking through a virtual enchanted forest. Who says fitness can't be magical?

The Case of the Confused Voice Assistant: I often laugh during class, when the instructor puts on her favorite loud track to a yoga meditation class.

Asking your voice assistant to play workout music and ending up with a symphony instead is part of the charm. Bonus points if you do squats to Beethoven.

From Sweatbands to Smart Bands: Once upon a time, fitness was about tracksuits and cassette players. Fast forward to today, and we've swapped those for moisture-wicking leggings and smartwatches that count every calorie, step, and heartbeat. Technology has revolutionized how we approach fitness, making it easier to track progress, stay motivated, and connect with others on the same journey.

Gearing Up with Fitness Tech: Technology doesn't just make fitness more efficient—it makes it more fun. Gadgets like fitness trackers, smartwatches, and heart rate monitors allow you to measure progress and set achievable goals.

Even if you are single or taking exercise by yourself there's an online fitness community out for you. Online fitness groups are the new coffee meets. Sharing tips, celebrating milestones, and maybe even engaging in a little friendly competition. It's all about staying connected while staying fit, especially with others. Try their routes or see what local events everyone is attending and arrange a meet-up. You will never be alone again.

Top Tech for Fitness

1. **Smartwatches:** Track steps, heart rate, and even sleep patterns.
2. **Fitness Apps:** From yoga to strength training, apps provide guided workouts.
3. **Wireless Earbuds:** Stream your favorite playlist or podcast while staying active.
4. **Video Platforms:** Follow fitness videos on YouTube or subscription services.
5. **Telehealth Wearables:** Devices that sync with apps to share health data with doctors.

Inspirational Story:
Hazel, 67, started using a fitness tracker to monitor her daily steps. "At first, 5,000 steps seemed impossible," she admits. "Now, I hit 10,000 most days without even trying—and the celebratory buzz it gives me feels like winning an award!"

Fun Task:
If you have a fitness tracker, set a step goal for the week and challenge yourself to beat it daily. No tracker? Use your phone's pedometer feature instead.

Dressing the (Techy) Part:
Tracksuits have come a long way since the 80s. Today's fitness wear combines functionality and flair, and the right outfit can boost both your confidence and performance.

Tips for Tech-Friendly Activewear

1. **Moisture-Wicking Fabrics:** Stay cool and dry during workouts.
2. **Leggings with Pockets:** Perfect for stashing your phone or keys.
3. **Reflective Gear:** Ideal for early morning or evening workouts.

4. **Smart Textiles:** Wearables that integrate tech like heart rate sensors.
5. **Wireless Fitness Accessories:** Like Bluetooth-enabled headphones for seamless activity.

Fun Task:
Raid your closet and find one outfit that makes you feel fabulous and functional for your next workout. Snap a selfie and rock your gear!

Apps to Keep You Moving: Fitness technology isn't always smooth sailing.

The Accidental Screenshot: Somehow, you've taken 15 photos of your wrist during your morning walk.

The Overachieving App: Your yoga app cheerfully suggests "advanced poses" that feel more like circus tricks.

Battery Anxiety: Nothing derails a good workout like a low-battery warning on your smartwatch. Solution? Always carry a portable charger—because fitness waits for no one. Fitness apps make it easy to work out at home, join virtual classes, or simply keep track of your progress. They're like having a personal trainer in your pocket—minus the hefty fees.

Staying Connected Through Fitness:
Fitness isn't just about physical health—it's also a social experience. Technology allows you to connect with friends, join virtual classes, and even compete in online challenges.

Ways to Use Tech for Social Fitness

1. **Virtual Classes:** Join live sessions through platforms like Zoom or Facebook Live.
2. **Fitness Challenges:** Compete with friends on step-count leaderboards.

3. **Social Media Groups:** Share your progress and cheer each other on.
4. **Wearable Tech Alerts:** Share activity achievements with friends via your devices.
5. **Streaming Workouts:** Follow along with fitness influencers or subscription services.

Staying Connected Through Fitness:
Fitness isn't just about physical health—it's also a social experience. Technology allows you to connect with friends, join virtual classes, and even compete in online challenges.

Fun Task:
Invite a friend to join you in a virtual fitness challenge or class this week. Share your progress and encourage each other to stay motivated.

Weekly Checklist: The Tech and Tracksuits Challenge

Ready to embrace fitness tech and trendy gear? Here's your 5-step challenge:

1. **Track Your Steps:** Use a pedometer or app to monitor daily activity.
2. **Try a New Fitness App:** Explore a guided workout or activity tracker.
3. **Dress the Part:** Wear a functional yet fashionable outfit for your next workout.
4. **Set a Tech Goal:** Whether it's steps, calories burned, or miles walked, aim to meet it by week's end.
5. **Share Your Progress:** Post a selfie or update in a fitness group to celebrate your achievements.

6. **Think comfortable:** staying cool or warm (seasons), snug fitting gear.
7. **Safety:** Pick routes and locations where you feel safe. Always tell someone your planned route and the approximate time you will be on your daily activity to a partner or friend. The park is always a great place if you feel good near a toilet, cafe, and other visitors in the park.
8. **Contact and Medical:** Information details in a waterproof pouch.

The Future of Fitness Tech

The possibilities are endless;

Augmented Reality Workouts: Imagine jogging through the streets of Paris while walking on your treadmill.

Smart Clothes: Coming soon to a closet near you: tracksuits that monitor your muscle activity and give real-time feedback.

Holographic Trainers: Why settle for a video when a virtual coach can appear in your living room to cheer you on?

A Day in the Life: Fitness Tech in Action

Here's how a tech-enhanced day might look:

Morning Walk: Slip on your GPS-enabled trainers and let them guide you on a scenic route.

Midday Yoga: Follow a guided class on your tablet, complete with calming visuals and real-time adjustments.

Evening Cool-Down: Your smartwatch suggests a stretching routine and tracks your progress while syncing calming music to your pace.

Final Humorous Anecdote:

Chris proudly told her granddaughter about her new smartwatch.

"It's amazing!" she said. "It buzzes when I sit too long, tracks my steps, and even gives me weather updates. Next thing you know, it'll tell me what's for dinner!"

Embracing the Change:

At 60+, you're not just keeping up with the times, you're redefining them. Tech and tracksuits are tools for living your best life, not just keeping up with trends. So strap on that smartwatch, zip up that chic tracksuit, and own your fitness journey with style, humor, and a touch of modern magic.

Conclusion: Teching It One Step at a Time

Technology and fitness gear have given us more tools than ever to stay active, connected, and stylish. Whether you're tracking your steps, joining a virtual class, or rocking a new workout outfit, it's all about finding what works for you.

It has taken me a few years to embrace gadgets and smart devices, it's an ongoing project. I seem to have more things to pack than ever before, crazy. I still enjoy the free no-backpack days!

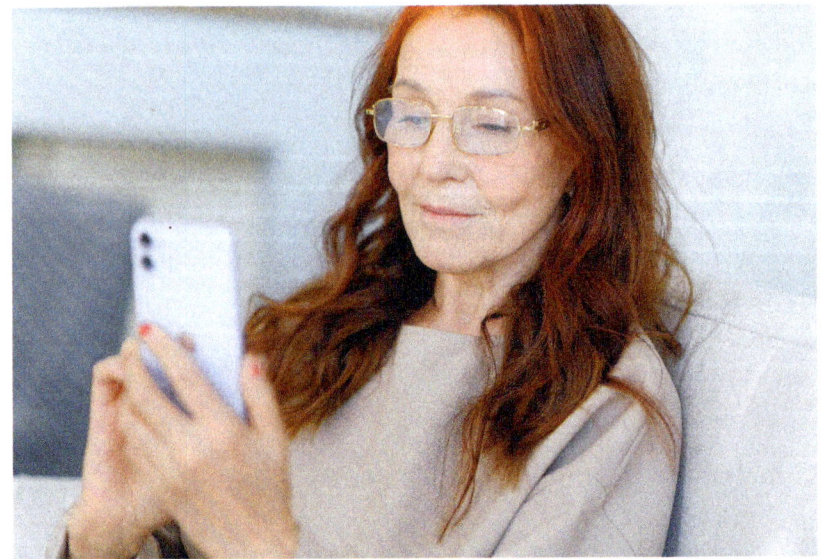

"Embracing the future: Discover the power of tech gadgets for fitness and safety."

Embrace the tech, rock the tracksuit, and show the world that fitness after 60 is as vibrant and exciting as ever. Let's tech it, one step at a time!

Rest Days and Naps: The Real MVPs

Your muscles need time to repair and grow, and your brain needs time to process how amazing you're becoming. Rest days aren't "lazy" days; they're productivity in disguise. Plus, a good nap can do wonders for your complexion, who doesn't want to wake up looking five years younger?

"Walking in the woods recharges your spirit—until you spot a squirrel and remember why you stick to city parks."

Let's talk about the unsung hero of fitness: rest. It's like the chocolate cake of workouts—everyone needs a slice.

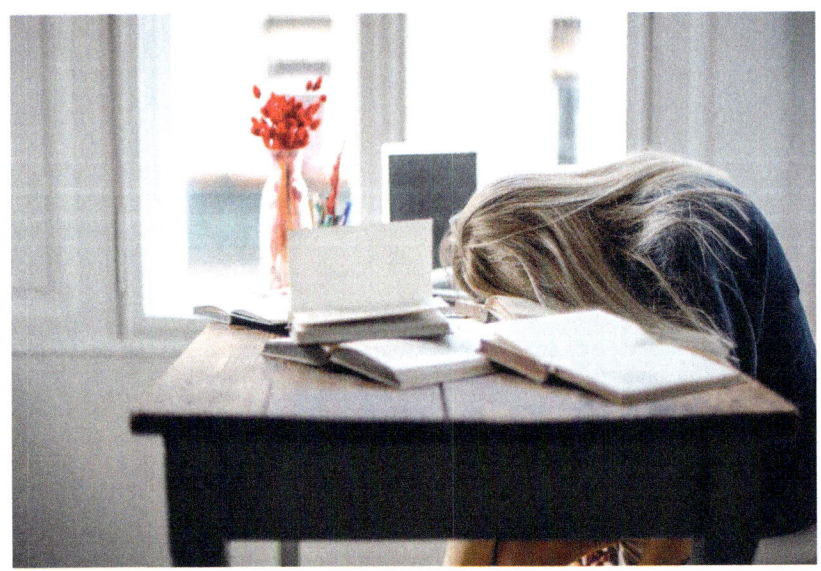

"Recharging for success: The art of napping enhances recovery, boosts productivity, and restores energy."

Why Recovery is Just as Important as Exercise

Your muscles need time to repair and grow, and your brain needs time to process how amazing you're becoming. Rest days aren't "lazy" days; they're productivity in disguise. Plus, a good nap can do wonders for your complexion, who doesn't want to wake up looking five years younger?

Some of us ladies will find the need to run, jog, or go to the gym on rest days. Just learn that the day after your training activity you will feel ready to get on with it, looking forward to your fitness days. I do have a day off every week. When I am training for a long race around week 12, naps become more important along with rest days.

If you are getting a cold, snuffling, or feeling rough then walk only. The best medicine ever for healing is outdoors in the fresh air. You do not need to stay indoors get outside and enjoy. It is best to stay away from crowds of other people in close confines if you are feeling down. It is all about keeping your immune system strong to fend off any incoming colds.

The Art of the Power Nap

The secret to a great nap is timing. Too short, and you're crankier than a cat in a bathtub. Too long, and you wake up wondering what year it is. The sweet spot? Twenty minutes. Just enough to recharge without slipping into "I'll sleep when I'm retired" mode.

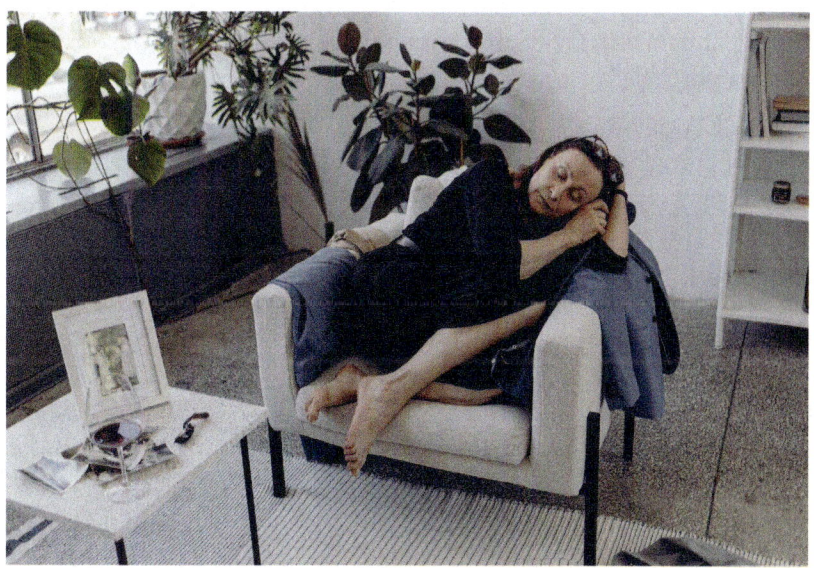

"Embrace rest without guilt: Find a comfortable spot to relax and recharge, instead of pretending you're not tired."

Nap Like a Pro—The Art of Rest Days:
Taking naps and enjoying rest days over 60 isn't just about recharging, it's an art form. At this stage in life, you've earned the right to embrace the glorious joys of doing nothing and call it self-care. Forget "lazy", you're conserving energy for the big moments, like a marathon shopping spree or dancing at a family wedding.

Margaret Thatcher, the UK Prime Minister was famous for taking short power naps to recharge. It is believed that ancient man would also take a power nap in the afternoons. For me, it is always around 2 pm and again around 9 pm then I am good to go until the early hours. Some of my best writing and creativity is in the early hours. It is a time when the phone doesn't ring. It's so peaceful everywhere. It is the best time to get my head in a good place to plan for the next day.

Recharge and Reboot:
Just like your phone, you work better after a little plug-in time. Except you're not staring at a wall socket, you're nestled into your favorite recliner, blanket at the ready.

Boost Your Mood:
A 20-minute nap can turn a cranky day into a cheerful one. Think of it as hitting the reset button with bonus dreams about winning the lottery.

Fuel for the Fun:
Whether it's grandkid adventures, a hobby marathon, or dominating trivia night, naps keep you ready to conquer life's most exciting challenges.

The Nap-O-Meter: Finding Your Perfect Snooze Style

Not all naps are created equal.
   Here's a guide to discovering what kind of napper you are:

1. The Power Nap (10-20 Minutes)
   Perfect for a quick pick-me-up. Just enough to refresh, not enough to confuse you about what year it is when you wake up.

2. The Classic Siesta (30-60 Minutes)
   A solid midday rest to recharge for the afternoon. Pairs well with a cup of tea and a guilt-free snack. That describes Me.

3. The "Accidental Couch Nap"
   Start with "I'm just going to close my eyes for a minute" and end with waking up to your favorite show's credits rolling. Bonus points if there's drool involved. I'm good at this one too around 9 pm. I start watching a movie then wake up just in time to see the ending and wonder what happened. My husband says when I declare I haven't seen a movie, he will say that was the one you fell asleep to last time!

4. The Luxury Nap (2 Hours or More)
   The kind of nap that says, "I've got nowhere to be, and I'm loving it." Warning: This may lead to wondering if it's still the same day.

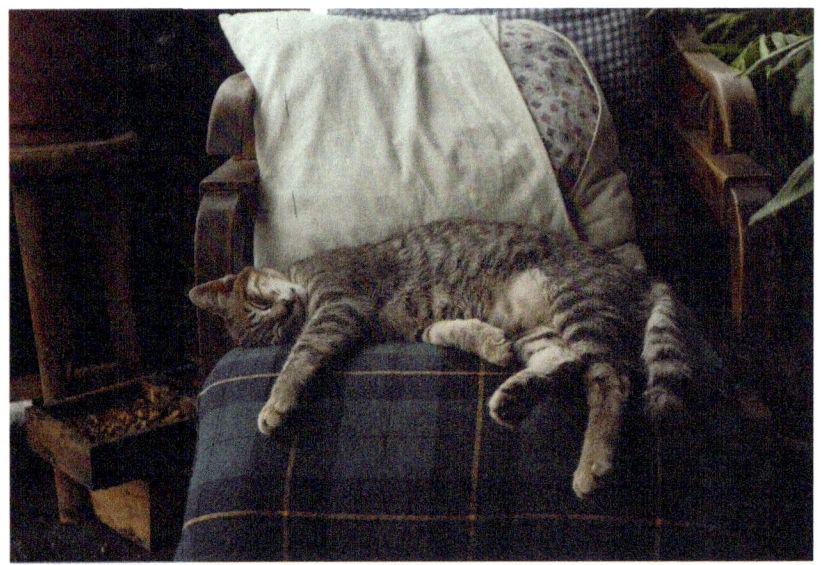

"Channel your inner cat: Master the art of relaxation and recharging, always ready to spring into action when needed."

Rest Days Are Not Lazy Days:
Let's debunk the myth: rest days aren't about doing nothing, they're about doing everything your body needs to feel amazing.

Stretching and Lounging: Call it "active relaxation." A little yoga followed by a long recline is peak balance.

Binge-Watching as Therapy: Who says catching up on your favorite show isn't a form of rest? Laughter counts as exercise, after all. I like this one.

Reading and Sipping: Whether it's a juicy novel or the crossword, engage your mind while your body chills.

The "I'll Just Rest My Eyes" Scenario:
You're halfway through a book just thinking, "I'll just rest my eyes for a second." Two hours later, you're drooling on the pages, and your tea is cold.

Over-committing to Relaxation:
"I'll relax all day tomorrow!" you promise. Then tomorrow arrives, and your to-do list guilt creeps in. Solution? Make the to-do list optional—except for naps.

The Battle of the Blanket Thief:
If you share a couch with a pet or partner, you know the struggle: they always seem to win the blanket tug-of-war. I dealt with that one because we have our huge comfy sofas to nap in. **Pro tip: get a decoy blanket for them to steal.**

Mastering the Art of Napping and Resting

Set the Mood:
Comfy clothes, a soft blanket, and maybe some calming music. Think spa vibes but with fewer cucumbers on your eyes. Works well at my weekly yoga class. Sharon, my teacher never minds the odd snort or snoring.

No Apologies:
You don't need to justify a nap or a lazy day to anyone. If someone questions it, simply reply, "I'm charging my life batteries."

Celebrate the Pause:
Rest isn't the absence of productivity, it's what makes productivity possible. So, savor it.

The Nap Hall of Fame: True Stories of Resting Glory

My best nap story was recently when I took an afternoon nap around 2 pm. I must have got into a deep sleep with the blinds drawn. When I woke up I got into a sudden panic as I believed it was early morning. I got into bed and saw that my husband, who prefers to take himself off to bed for his afternoon nap, was still in bed. I got into bed as he stirred saying is it that late. I replied no I cannot believe I slept on the sofa all night. I won't feel fantastic today, still I can still grab an hour before getting up.

As I write it is winter happening to me last month it was already dark. My husband said I better get up. I said it's a bit early for you. He replied what time do you think it is? I said 6 am isn't it looking at him. He laughed saying can't wait to tell the kids! Feeling embarrassed it dawned on me that I had only napped a few hours not all night! Oh dear. I have not been able to live that down with the kids or my husband. He loves to tell everyone.

If that could be you, set the alarm to save disorientation and time travel.

I've spun it around to become a professional couch napper, known for my ability to snooze through an entire movie marathon, and still claim I've "watched the whole thing."

Laughing Through the Laziness:

Let's embrace the funny side of rest days: When your family calls you out for napping too much, remind them, "Even superheroes take breaks between saving the world."

Ever tried to nap, only for your pet to demand attention? You're not resting, you're providing warmth and comfort to your fur overlord, my

5 cats fight for my lap, and shoulders and jump on my back, as they have done on many occasions as I write this book for my sole personal groomer's attention.

Did you forget to turn off your phone and get startled by a ringtone mid-nap? Instant heart rate boost, who needs cardio? Place your phone in airplane mode for naps.

Napping Conclusions: Nap Without Guilt, Rest With Pride

Rest isn't just a luxury, it's a necessity. Rest keeps you sharp, energized, and ready to tackle whatever comes next. So fluff your pillow, embrace the snooze, and remember: there's nothing lazy about listening to what your body and soul need.

And when you wake up, refreshed and revitalized, feel free to say, "I'm not lazy, I'm just this good at self-care."

Walking in the Woods: Nature's Perfect Rest Day

If you don't feel like a nap, take a relaxing energizing walk.

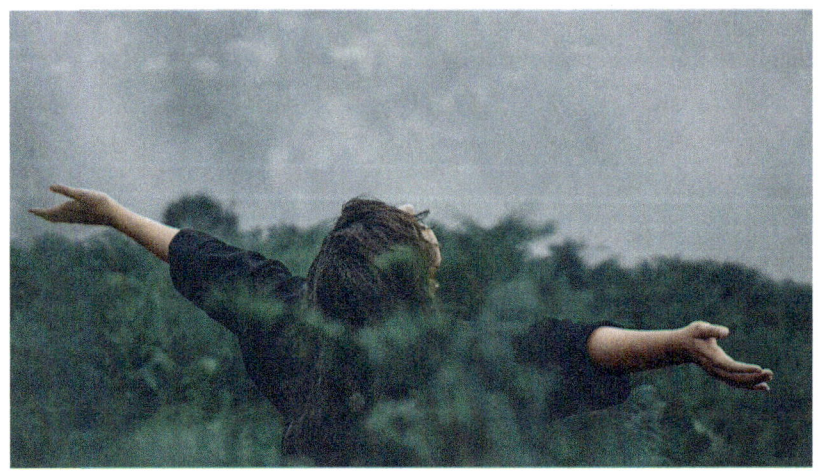

Embracing nature's healing power, let the outdoors restore your energy on recovery days.

For those of us who find solace in the outdoors, rest days aren't about napping or lounging, they're about strolling. Walking in the woods is the ultimate reset button.

The rustle of leaves underfoot, the whisper of the wind through the trees, and the occasional chatter of birds create a symphony of calm that recharges your mind, body, and spirit. It's not just a walk; it's a journey into stillness, where the worries of the world fade into the background, and the simple joy of being alive takes center stage. Whether it's a brisk hike or a leisurely wander, the woods offer a sanctuary where every step feels like a step toward wholeness. Do what makes you happy and enjoy your rest days.

Laughing Through It All-The Power of Humor After 60+

Who says fitness has to be all grit and no giggles? Exercise isn't just about reps, sets, and serious faces, it's about enjoying yourself and finding joy in the journey. Laughter is a secret weapon, turning challenges into triumphs and making every workout brighter.

In this chapter, we'll explore how humor and playfulness can enhance your fitness routine, reduce stress, and keep you coming back for more. From funny mishaps at Zumba to the unexpected hilarity of a yoga class, you'll discover why laughter is the best workout buddy.

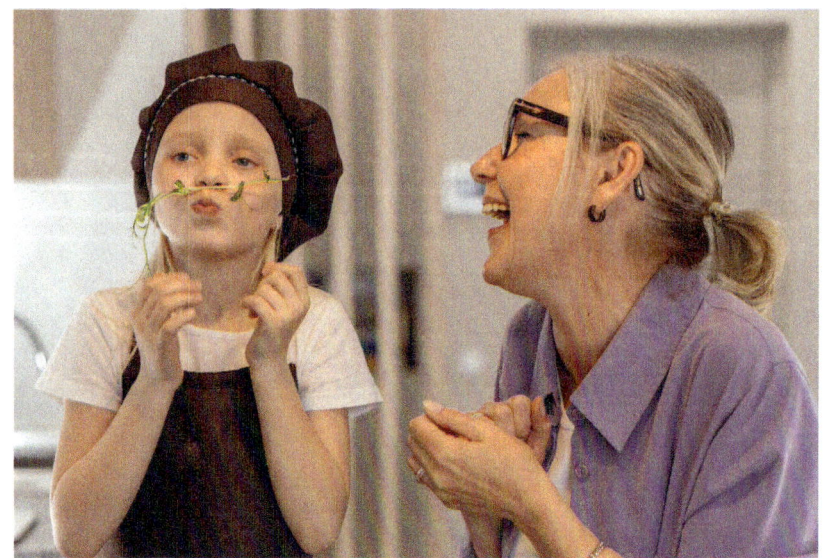

A moment of joy reminds us that laughter is essential to our well-being and fitness

"Laughter is the best exercise, it tightens your abs, lifts your mood, and won't make you sore the next day."

The Healing Power of Laughter

Laughter isn't just fun—it's good for your health. Studies show that a good laugh can:

- Boost your immune system.
- Increase blood flow.
- Release endorphins (those feel-good hormones).
- Relax your muscles for up to 45 minutes.
- Combine that with the benefits of exercise, and you've got a recipe

for total wellness.

Top Benefits of Laughing While Exercising:

- **Stress Relief:** Laughter reduces cortisol, the stress hormone.
- **Core Workout:** Belly laughs engage your abdominal muscles.
- **Improved Endurance:** A good mood can help you push through tough workouts.
- **Social Connection:** Sharing laughs builds bonds with your fitness buddies.
- **Enhanced Enjoyment:** You're more likely to stick with activities that make you happy.

Inspirational Story:

Pauline, 72, joined a laughter yoga class and never looked back. "At first, I felt silly," she says. "But by the end, I was laughing so hard my cheeks hurt—and I couldn't wait to come back."

Fun Task:

Schedule a "silly workout" this week—whether it's laughter yoga, a goofy dance session, or trying a TikTok challenge with friends.

Turning Mishaps into Memories:

Let's face it: exercise doesn't always go as planned. From slipping on a yoga mat to tripping over a jump rope, fitness bloopers are inevitable. But instead of getting frustrated, why not laugh it off?

If I had to choose, the most common embarrassment that we've all faced would be to break wind whilst bending over without any warning. That's the life we have all been there at some stage!

Common Workout Blunders (and How to Laugh at Them):

The Misstep: Missed a Zumba step? Keep moving and call it "freestyle."

Wardrobe Malfunctions: A too-loose waistband can turn into a hilarious tale.

Unintentional Sounds: Yoga class is full of surprises, sometimes audible ones.

Equipment Failures: If the treadmill ejects you, make it part of the routine!

Forgetfulness: Showing up to swim class without a swimsuit is just another reason to chuckle.

Humorous Anecdote:

For me, it was someone stepping on my shoe heel at the start of the Valencia Marathon as the thousands ran over the line. I was dodging runners and walkers chasing my trainer as it was being kicked further away from my grasp. Luckily a runner had seen my distress and kicked the shoe to one side to save me from getting trampled on literally to put my shoe back on in a safe place. I had to laugh later as my husband and coach said great that slowed you from setting off too fast as I normally do, we both laughed later.

Fun Task: Share a funny fitness story with a friend or post it online. You'll laugh, and so will they!

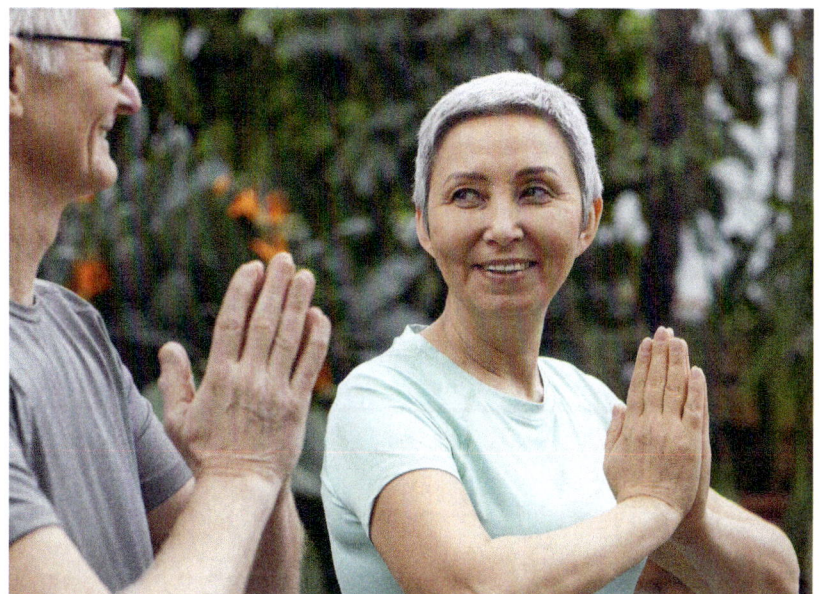

"Finding joy in the flow: Laughter and connection on the mat are as healing as the practice itself."

Laughter is and always will be the best form of therapy ~ **Audrey Hepburn** Actress

Group Classes and Giggles:
 Working out in a group often leads to shared laughs, whether it's over confusing instructions or the collective struggle of a tough class.

Funny Fitness Group Moments:

- **Synchrony Struggles:** That moment when everyone goes left, except you.
- **Unintended Comedy:** An instructor's quirky phrases can become inside jokes.

- **Competitive Banter:** Friendly teasing adds a spark to any class.
- **Unlikely Pairings:** Seeing your serious neighbor ace a silly dance move is priceless.
- **Shared Relief:** The collective groan at the end of a tough set is oddly bonding.

Inspirational Story:

Beth, 68, joined a seniors' kickboxing class and found herself laughing more than punching. "We weren't exactly fast or fierce," she says, "but every time someone missed the bag, we'd crack up. It became the highlight of my week."

Fun Task:

Sign up for a new group class this week—bonus points if it sounds a little out of your comfort zone.

Laughing at Yourself (And Loving It):

Fitness isn't about perfection. It's about showing up, trying your best, and sometimes looking a little silly in the process. Embracing those moments can make your journey more enjoyable and less intimidating.

Ways to Laugh at Yourself:

- **Celebrate the "Fails":** Every stumble is a step toward growth.
- **Keep Perspective**: Remember, everyone starts somewhere.
- **Find the Fun:** Treat each challenge like a game.
- **Share the Humor:** Post a lighthearted update about your fitness adventures.
- **Remind Yourself Why You're Doing It:** A smile makes it all worthwhile.

Let's Face it Girls: life gives us plenty to laugh about at our age and practice your pelvic floor muscles holding it all in! From the joys of trying to remember where you put your glasses (hint: they're on your head) to the hilarity of tech mishaps with your smartphone, humor is everywhere if you know where to look.

They say laughter is the best medicine, and in our 60s, it's practically a superpower. A good laugh doesn't just lighten the mood, it makes every challenge feel just a little more manageable. After all, if you can chuckle at life's absurdities, you're already winning.

Why Laughter is Your Fountain of Youth
  It Keeps You Healthy:
  Laughter reduces stress, boosts your immune system, and even gives your abs a mini workout. Who needs crunches when a good belly laugh can do the job?
  It Builds Connections:
  Sharing a laugh with friends, family, or even strangers strengthens bonds. It's a universal language that says, "We're in this together."
  So go ahead, laugh through it all, every wobble, every stumble, every funny face. Your fitness journey will be lighter, brighter, and infinitely more enjoyable.

Finding Humor in Everyday Life:

1. The "Senior Moment" Chronicles
  Misplacing your keys, forgetting names, or walking into a room and asking, "Why am I here?" These moments are comedy gold. Why stress when you can laugh?
  Pro Tip: Write down your funniest "senior moments" and turn them

into a stand-up routine for family gatherings.

2. Technology Troubles

Ever tried explaining to your phone's voice assistant that you want "Directions to Target," not "Recipes for Tarts"? Technology is a treasure trove of hilarity.

Bonus: Pretend your grandkids are your IT department, it's a surefire way to confuse them and make them laugh.

3. The Body's Betrayal (or Is It?)

Achy knees? A back that makes noises like bubble wrap? Laugh it off! Every snap, crackle, and pop is just your body's way of singing the song of experience.

How to Infuse More Laughter into Your Life.

Watch or Listen to Comedy: Whether it's a classic sitcom, a stand-up special, or a funny podcast, surround yourself with things that make you smile.

Embrace Playfulness: Channel your inner childs play a board game, tell a silly joke, or try karaoke. Who cares if you're off-key?

Laugh at Yourself: When life gets ridiculous, lean into it. Spilled coffee? Dropped the remote? Forgot what day it is. It's all part of the grand comedy show.

The Joy of Shared Laughter: One of the best things about laughter is that it's contagious.

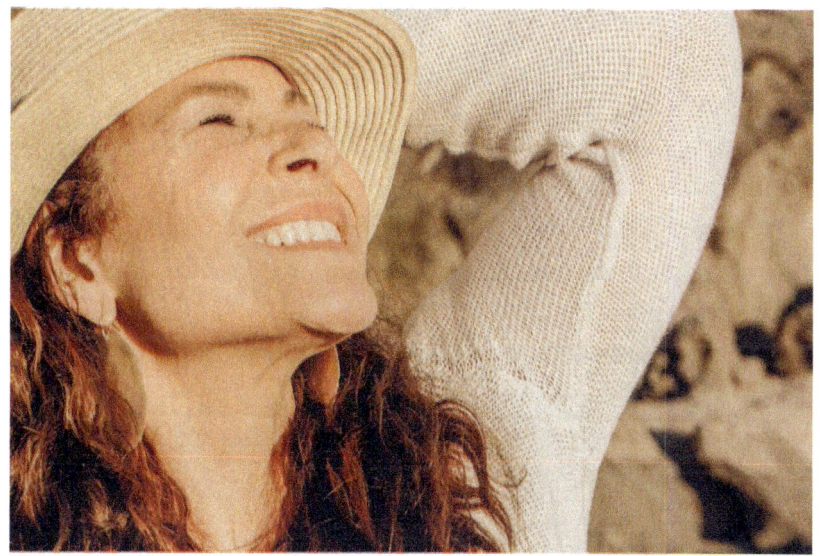

"Radiating joy: Embracing the beauty of life with a heart full of gratitude and a smile to match."

Here are ways to spread the joy:

With Friends: Share funny stories, play charades, or host a comedy movie night.

With Family: Let the grandkids teach you TikTok dances—it's guaranteed to end in giggles.

In the Community: Join a laughter yoga class (yes, it's a thing!) or attend local comedy shows.

Fun Task: Take a "post-workout selfie" this week and send it to a friend with a funny caption.

The Science of Laughing More: Studies show that even fake laughter can trigger the same benefits as the real thing. So, the next time you're feeling down, try forcing a laugh, it might just turn into the real deal. Bonus points if you do it in front of a mirror for maximum hilarity.

Humor as a Coping Tool:

Life isn't always sunshine and rainbows, but humor can help you weather the storms. Here's how:

In Health Challenges: Finding something to laugh about even during tough times can lighten the emotional load and remind you of your resilience.

In Relationships: Humor can diffuse tension, smooth over disagreements, and keep your bonds strong.

In Aging: Wrinkles? Call them laughter lines. Slower pace? Say you're just taking the scenic route.

Laugh Your Way Through It:

Humor is the ultimate life hack. It's free, endlessly renewable and available to everyone. So, embrace the funny side of life, tell a corny joke, laugh at your quirks, and remember: the secret to staying young at heart is to not take yourself too seriously.

Here's to laughing through it all—because over 60, you've got more reasons to smile than ever, who cares what others think of you conserving yourself and your energies for healthy longevity?

The Weekly Laughter Challenge

Ready to add some giggles to your routine? Here's your 5-step challenge:

- **Try a Silly Workout:** Dance, laugh, or join a goofy fitness class;
- **Embrace the Bloopers:** Laugh at any missteps and keep going;
- **Find a Workout Buddy:** Share the joy (and the jokes);
- **Tell a Funny Story:** Relive a fitness blooper with friends and
- **Celebrate the Fun:** Keep a journal of your happiest fitness

moments.

In the sweetness of friendship let there be laughter and sharing of pleasures. For in the dew of little things the heart finds its morning and is refreshed. ~ **Khalil Gibran**

The taking of this photo with my group had to be taken a few times, due to laughing. Some of us; mainly me, laughing so much I missed my camera action jump shot!

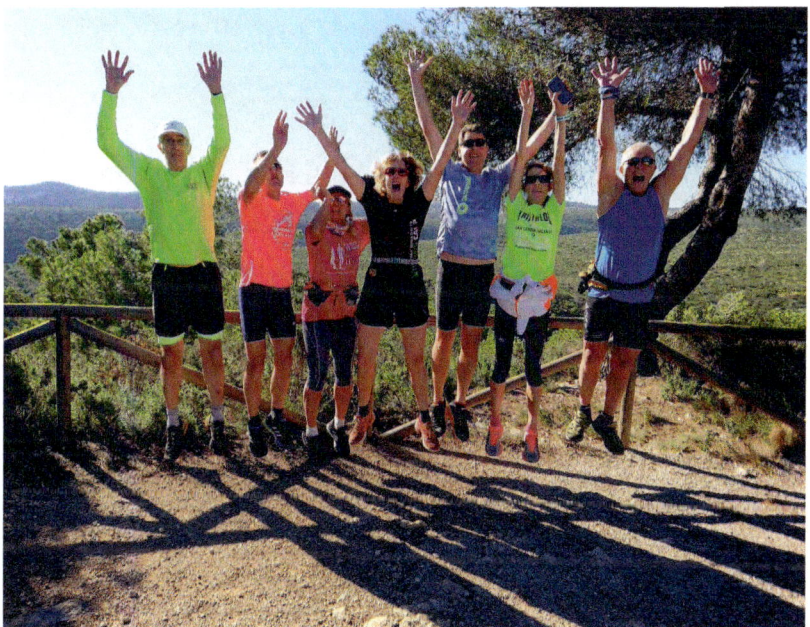

"Leaping into life: Celebrating fitness, friendship, and the pure joy of living with laughter and energy!"

Conclusion: Laugh It Out, Sweat It Out:

Fitness is a serious business, but it doesn't have to be somber. When you find joy and humor in your workouts, you're not just improving your body, you're lifting your spirit.

Tell a corny joke, my husband has no idea how he remembers them, but he has always made me laugh, that's a great attribute to have in any relationship, we do laugh. Just laugh at your quirks, and remember the secret to staying young at heart is to never take yourself too seriously. Here's to laughing through it all because, over 60, you've got more reasons to smile than ever.

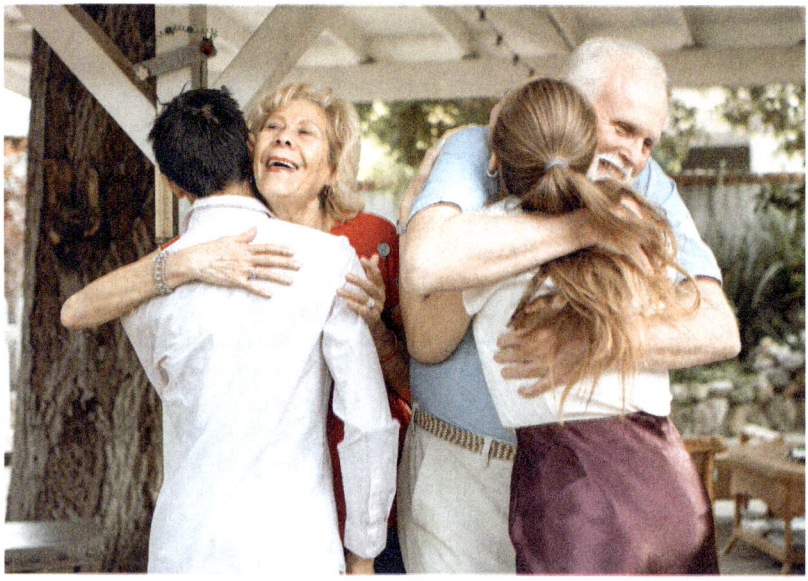

"Heart full, smiles wide: Cherishing the love and laughter that only family can bring."

Family gatherings always make me laugh being with friends and socializing. Laughter is a natural medicine, we need more of.

Your Fitness Legacy: Inspiring the Next Generation

In this chapter, we'll reflect on the journey you've taken so far, celebrate your achievements, and look ahead to what's possible. From creating bucket lists to finding a fresh purpose and getting fit, you'll see that the story of your life is far from over, it's just getting exciting. It's in your hands, you decide.

Life After 60 Celebrating Strength and Spirit

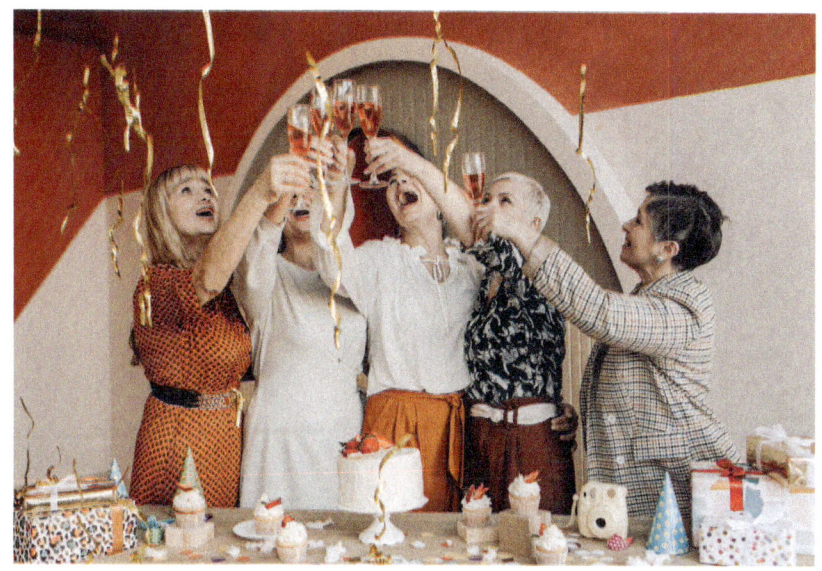

Cheers to another beautiful year: Celebrating life and friendship

"Life at 60+ isn't about slowing down, it's about speeding up the fun and coasting into joy."
To Be Continued

The Next Chapter Begins

Reaching 60 isn't the end of the book, it's the start of a thrilling new chapter. Think of it as a "choose your own adventure" story, where you're in the driver's seat, deciding what comes next. Whether it's exploring new hobbies, staying active, or discovering hidden talents, life after 60 is all about embracing what makes you feel alive. This is the time to embrace every aspect of your strength: physical, emotional, and spiritual.

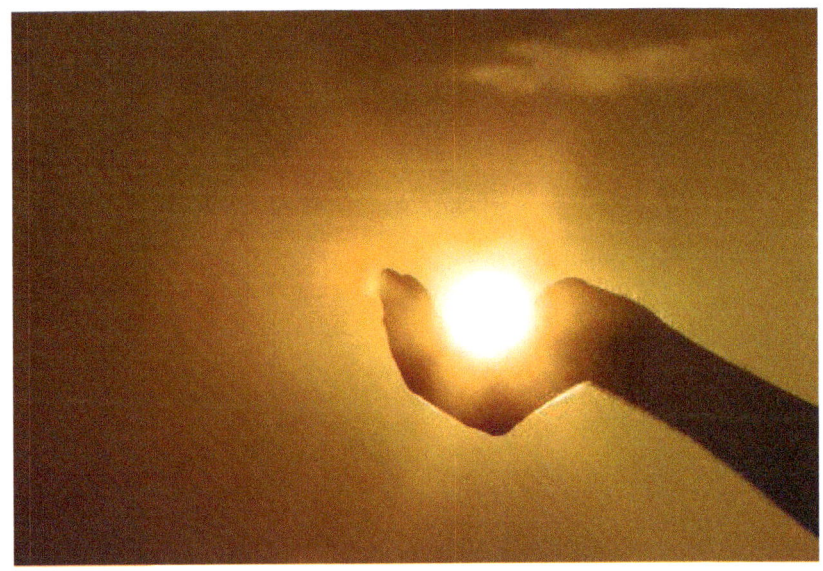

The Art of Saying Yes, I Can Do It

Redefining 60: The world has changed. At 60, you're not "over the hill", it's the new 50 you're standing at the summit, looking out at all the possibilities ahead.

Want to travel the world? Go for it.

Thinking of picking up a new hobby? Why not? Do that skydive or abseil down a building. Want to compete in a triathlon just to prove you can? You're unstoppable.

The Strength of Saying Yes:
  Yes to Adventure:
   Whether it's hiking, dancing, or learning to salsa, saying yes opens doors to new experiences.

Yes to Self-Care:
Strength isn't just about action it's about knowing when to rest, recharge, and take care of yourself.

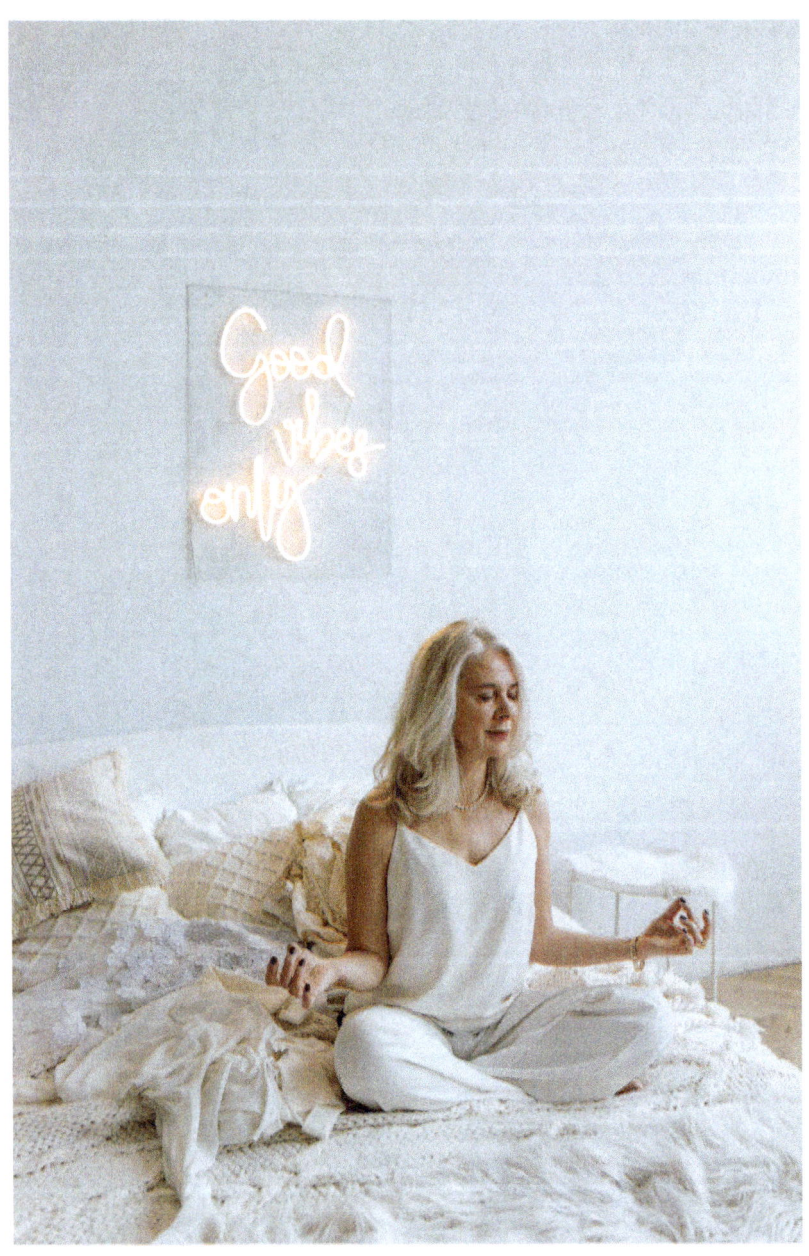

Be an inspirational role model for other women as the only time we have is right now
cciv

Yes to Fun:

Laughter isn't just good for the soul; it's a workout for the abs. Find reasons to smile every day you've earned it.

The Spirit of Giving Back

Strength also means sharing your gifts with others. Whether it's mentoring, volunteering, or simply being a source of wisdom for friends and family, your impact is immeasurable.

The joy of family and friends, who play such a big role in supporting all you do, and the ones who turn up on event day rain or sun, and sponsor all your beneficial community work. I delivered four thousand leaflets to homes on foot over a few days. I got paid for my time. For me, it was one huge fitness workout with miles covered and a good service for the local community too. Look to combine your workouts.

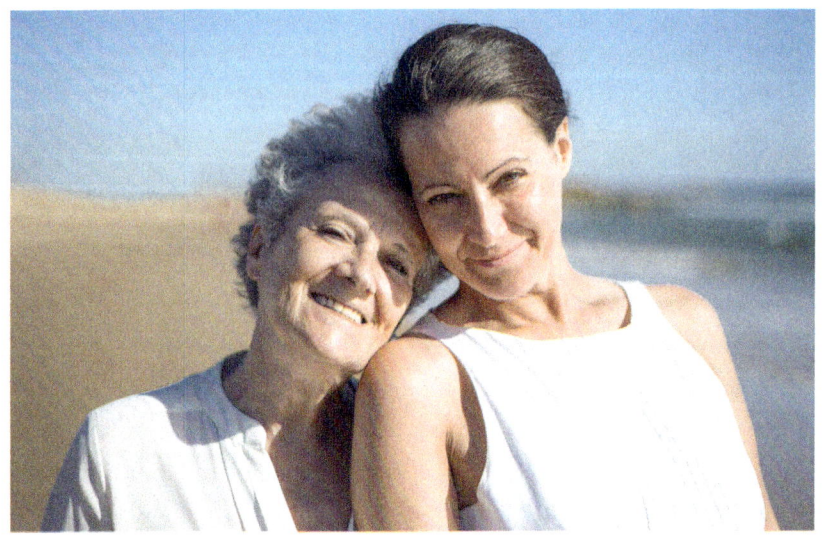

Dream it, do it: Inspiring adventures and unforgettable moments for the ultimate bucket list journey.

A 60+ Bucket List (Just for Fun):

Travel to a Dream Destination: Paris? Machu Picchu? A cozy cabin in the woods? Go where your heart leads.

Give yourself a special shopping day treat to get prepared. You will look and feel amazing and ready to start.

Try a New Sport or Activity: Kayaking, painting, stand-up paddle boarding what's stopping you?

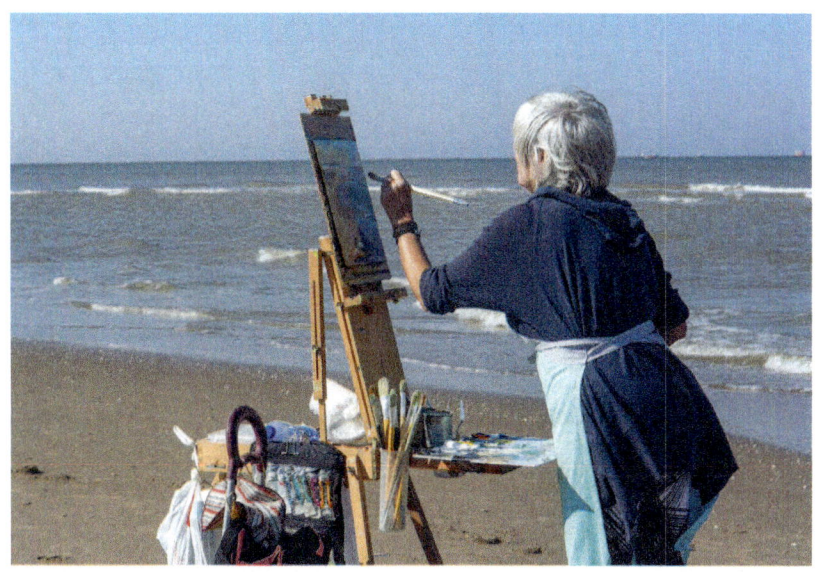

Embracing Creativity because it's never to start to start something new

Throw a "Life is Amazing" Party: Celebrate yourself and the incredible journey you've
  Had so far.
  Write Your Story: Share your adventures, wisdom, and laughter whether it's for your family or the world.

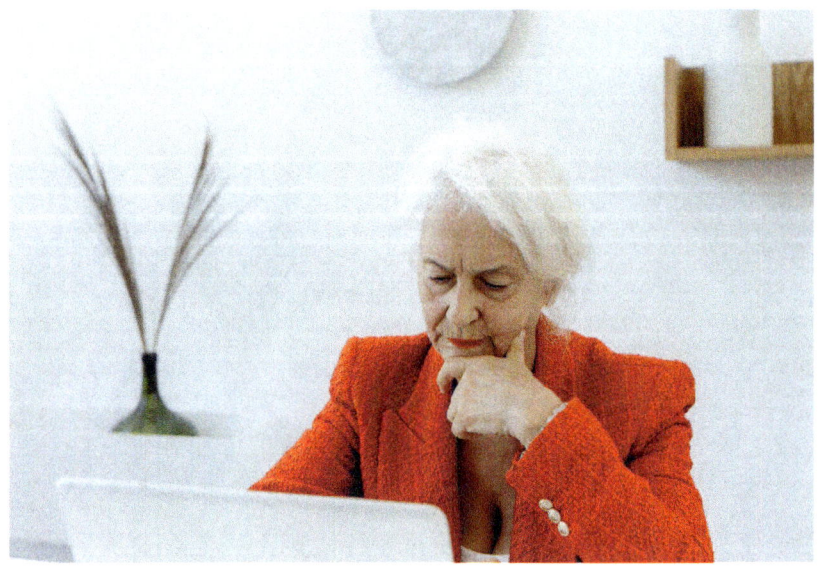

Learn Something New: A language, a musical instrument, or even how to make the perfect soufflé.

This chapter of life isn't about what you've left behind; it's about what's to come if you plan it. First, you need to get a basic level of fitness to start your new exciting life.

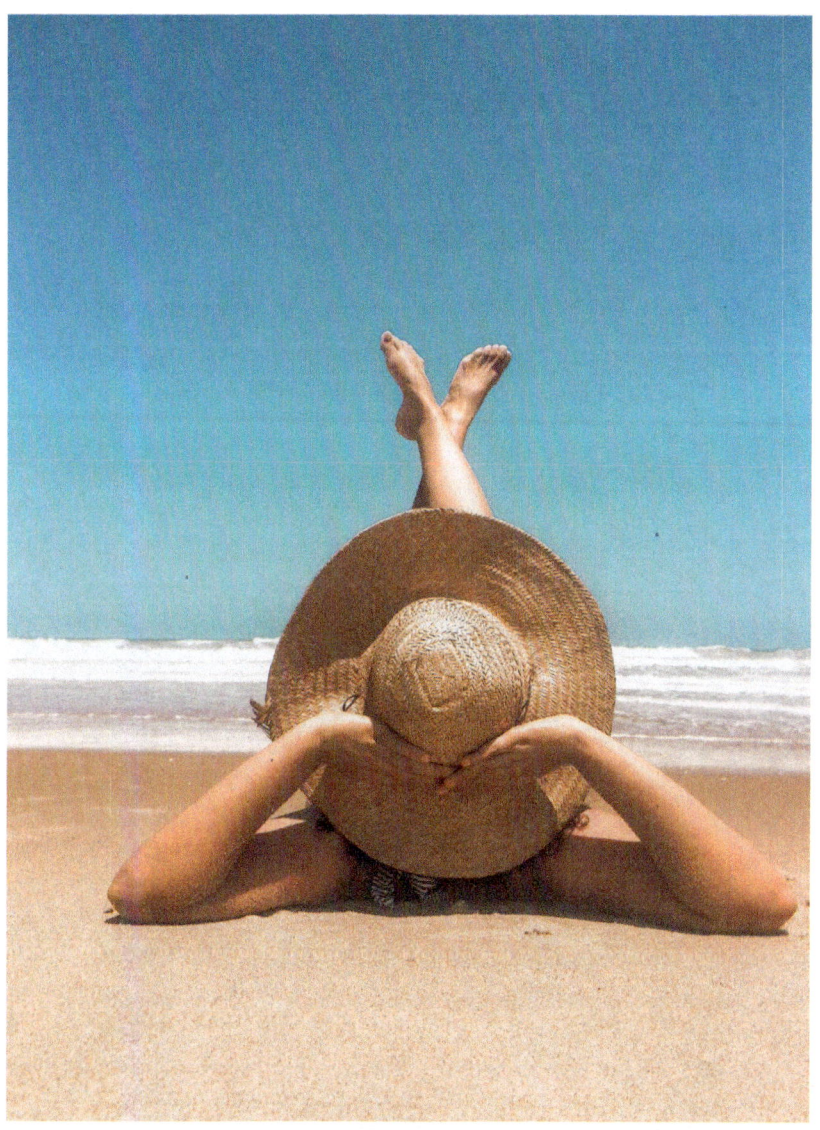

When in doubt travel

So here's to you dancing in the rain, laughing until your sides hurt, and living each day with real purpose.

I remember when my daughter bought me a T-shirt for my 60th birthday that read, *"Vintage, but still running."* I said thank you, "It's not just a slogan it's my new motto!" yeah let's go.

Reflecting on the Journey So Far

Before diving into what's next, it's important to take a moment to look back and appreciate how far you've come. Reflecting on your fitness journey, lifestyle changes, and personal growth can inspire you to keep moving forward.

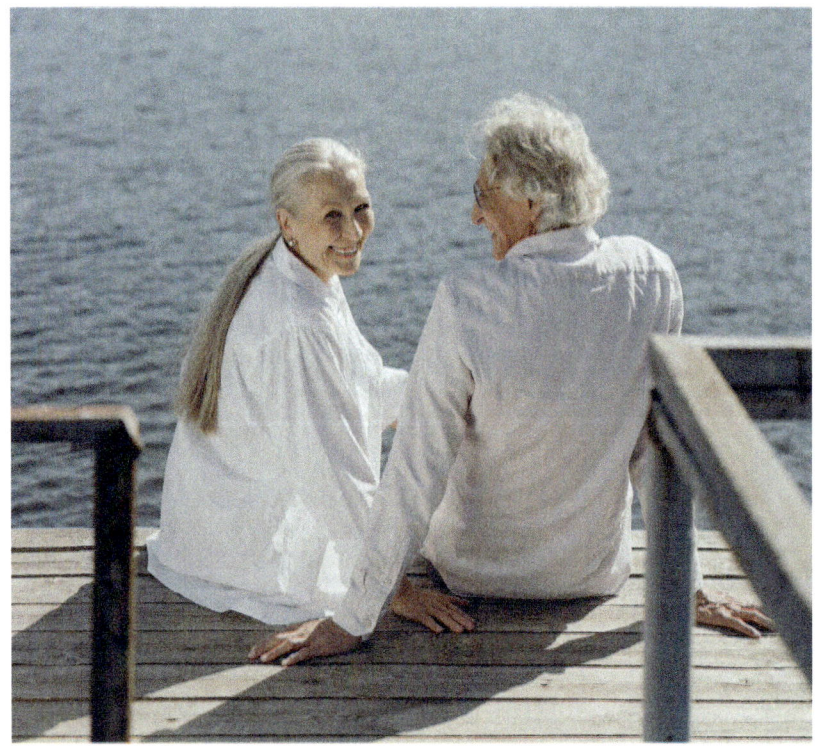

Questions To Ask Yourself

1. **What fitness goals have I achieved?** Celebrate your wins!
2. **What new activities or habits have I discovered?** Maybe you've fallen in love with yoga or started a walking group.
3. **How has my mindset shifted?** Fitness is as much about mental strength as physical strength.
4. **What challenges have I overcome?** Recognize your resilience.
5. **What's been the most fun?** Joy is a key ingredient in staying motivated.

Inspirational Story:

Shirley, 67, reflected on her first 5K race. "I was the last to finish, but I got the loudest cheers," she says. "That moment reminded me that it's never too late to try something new."

Fun Task:

Write a letter to your younger self, sharing the wisdom and experiences you've gained in the past year. Keep it as a reminder of how amazing you are.

Humorous Anecdote:

Georgia started journaling her fitness journey but kept getting sidetracked by doodling. "Turns out, my stick figures are doing better yoga poses than I am!"

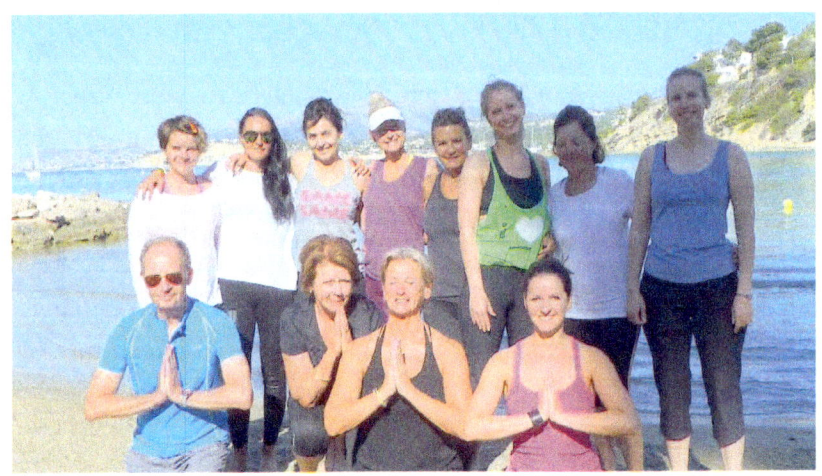

Meet Regularly for class and be missed by the group to stay on track

Create Your Fitness Bucket List

A bucket list isn't just for big life goals, it's perfect for fitness too. It's about setting fun, challenging, or slightly outrageous goals that keep you motivated and curious.

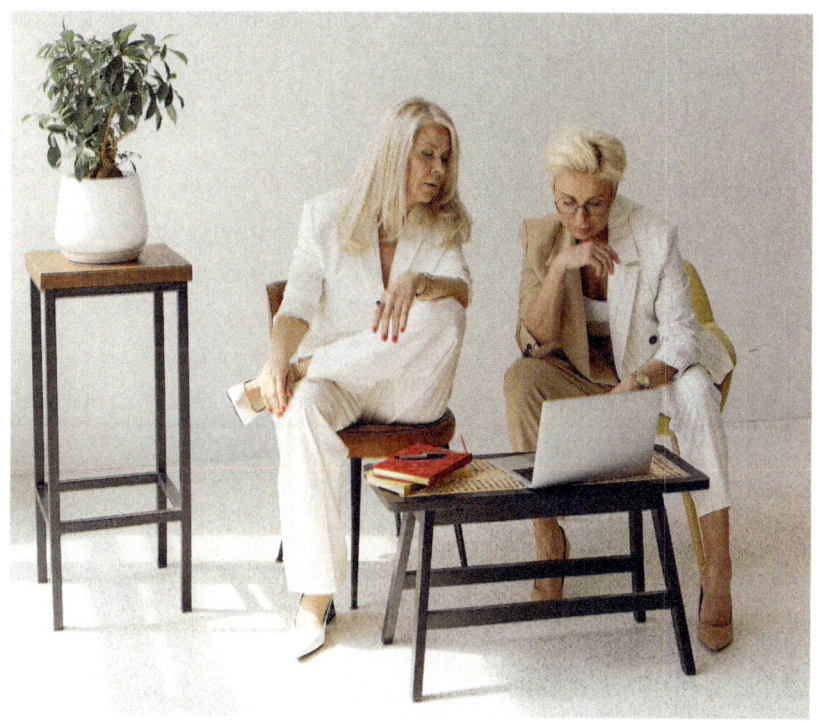

Success Loves Planning

Fitness Bucket List Ideas:

1. **Try a New Sport:** Archery? Kayaking? Something you've never tried before.
2. **Attend a Fitness Retreat:** Combine travel with wellness always or a hotel gym.
3. **Master a New Skill:** From tai chi to trail walking, the possibilities are endless.
4. **Complete a Fun Run:** Think charity races or themed 5km with costumes.

5. **Hit a Personal Best:** Whether it's lifting heavier, running faster, or stretching further.

Inspirational Story:

Helen, 72, set a goal to learn salsa dancing. "I thought my feet would never cooperate," she laughs, "but now I can't stop dancing even in the kitchen!"

Fun Task:

Start a fitness bucket list with at least five items. Share your list with a friend or family member who might want to join you.

Humorous Anecdote:

Beatrice added "skydiving yoga" to her bucket list, then realized it wasn't a real thing. "Guess I'll stick to Warrior Pose *on the ground*," she joked.

Embracing New Passions and Hobbies

Fitness isn't just about traditional workouts, it's about staying active in ways that bring you joy. Life after 60 is the perfect time to dive into hobbies that get your body moving and your heart singing.

Active Hobbies to Explore:

1. **Gardening:** Great for your muscles and your mood.
2. **Dancing:** Whether solo in your living room or at a class, it's pure fun.
3. **Cycling:** Enjoy the outdoors and relive the carefree joy of childhood rides.
4. **Photography Walks:** Combine exercise with creativity.
5. **Volunteer Work**: Activities like park clean-ups or dog walking

keep you moving.

Inspirational Story:
Barbara, 62, started leading walking tours of her city. "It's a workout and a chance to meet new people," she says. "Plus, I've learned more about my hometown than I ever knew!"

Fun Task:
Choose one new hobby to try this month. Bonus points if it involves movement!

Humorous Anecdote:
I took up archery with my husband as a new hobby. "Let's just say the arrows missed and landed everywhere for my patient instructor who spends more time picking them off the ground for me. I shout "Thank you keep going you need the exercise, he laughs but I'm having a blast!"

Looking Ahead with Confidence:
The best part of life after 60? You've got the wisdom and confidence to tackle whatever comes next. Setting realistic goals and staying open to new opportunities ensures that your story continues to evolve in exciting ways.

Tips for Moving Forward:

1. **Set SMART Goals:** Specific, Measurable, Achievable, Relevant, and Time-bound.
2. **Stay Curious:** Never stop exploring new ideas, places, and experiences.
3. **Prioritize Wellness:** Fitness, nutrition, and mental health go hand in hand.
4. **Find Your Community:** Surround yourself with supportive, like-minded people.
5. **Celebrate Yourself:** Every day is an opportunity to feel proud of

who you are.

Inspirational Story:

Helen started an over 60 hiking group that now boasts over 20 members. "We call ourselves the 'Silver Steppers,' and we've climbed hills I never thought I could," she says. We always spend all our walking journeys discussing the next walking holiday rather than all the other expats talking about their medicines, dodgy hips, and next doctor appointments. Life is too short, do what makes you happy, but keep moving.

Fun Task:

Write down three goals you want to achieve in the next year fitness-related or otherwise. Keep them visible as a daily reminder.

Humorous Anecdote:

I decided to try paddle boarding early one morning when the sea was calm in Spain. I had often seen so many out, it looked fantastic. I stopped that day on a conscious level and thought to myself that one day I would have a go at that. No will I do it, today is the day to get it booked. I have a can-do now attitude why wait now? It was brilliant fun. I did spend more time in the water, getting back up. At least I stayed cool.

Weekly Checklist: The "Life After 60" Challenge

Here's your 5-step challenge to kick-start the next chapter of your fitness journey:

1. **Reflect:** Spend 10 minutes journaling about your fitness achievements.
2. **Bucket List:** Add at least five fun fitness goals to your list.

3. **Try Something New:** Pick one activity you've never done before and give it a shot.
4. **Connect:** Join a class, group, or online community to share your journey.
5. **Celebrate:** Treat yourself to something special—because you've earned it!

Conclusion: The Story Continues

Turning 60 isn't a finish line, it's the start of an exciting new race. The adventures laughs, and milestones ahead are waiting for you to grab them with both hands. You will never retire from life, only your past career and work. It is truly your time now. Plan as you did when you started all those years ago. Set your daily goals, and fill them with joy, movement, and meaningful experiences. Just like when you were younger and dreams felt endless, it's time to dream again—this time with the wisdom of knowing what truly matters.

Pack more in these next years than you did when you were younger or bringing up the family. **Have your best life right now starting today.**

Final Humorous Anecdote:

At nearly 65, I'm sounding like a child who wants to be 5 and says they are four and a half proudly, I'm not slowing down I'm just picking up speed in a lane of my own. Watch out, world!"

Life after 60 is about more than staying fit; it's about thriving, laughing, and making every moment count. So keep moving, keep smiling, and remember: the best is yet to come. Time to misbehave.

Your Turn to Shine!

Congratulations, you've made it to the end of this journey, what an adventure we've had together! From neon leggings to belly laughs, from mindful stretching to the occasional cheeky nap, I hope this book has left you feeling inspired, empowered, and ready to embrace fitness and vitality in your unique way.

If this book made you smile, gave you a new perspective, or convinced you to take your first bold step (or stretch!)—I'd love to hear about it. Reviews are the lifeblood of authors like me, and your thoughts help others discover and enjoy this book too.

Please take a moment to leave a review on the platform where you purchased this book. Your feedback not only means the world to me but might inspire someone else to start their fitness journey.

Please share this book with a friend, workout buddy, or neighbor's dog walker. After all, fitness and laughter are always better when shared!

Thank you for being part of this journey. Here's to staying fabulous, fit, and full of life at any age!

With gratitude,
Amanda xxx

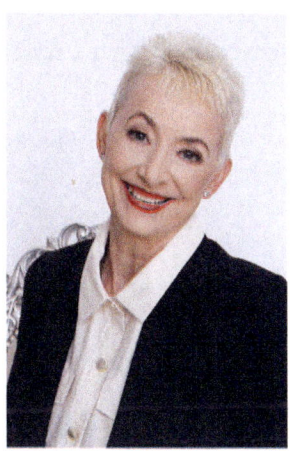

About the Author

Amanda Fletcher is a passionate advocate for health, wellness, and fitness, with a focus on empowering senior women to lead vibrant, fulfilling lives. At 64, Amanda embodies the transformative power of movement, proving that fitness is about more than physical activity—it's about nurturing the soul. She is an international Masters GB athlete and winner of many races including endurance mountain trail running.

Amanda also created yoga and running retreats in Spain, designed to help women recover from corporate burnout. Drawing on her expertise in mindful training, diet, and yoga, she inspires others with practical tools for transformation.

Since her spiritual awakening in 2012, Amanda has embraced writing as an intuitive outlet and a way to help others blossom in life. Her book, *Fitness for Senior Women Over 60,* was inspired by requests from other women seeking guidance. For Amanda, a book is the perfect way to combine her love of writing with her mission to encourage women over

50 and 60 years to rediscover their inner strength and embrace life with renewed energy.

Printed in Great Britain
by Amazon